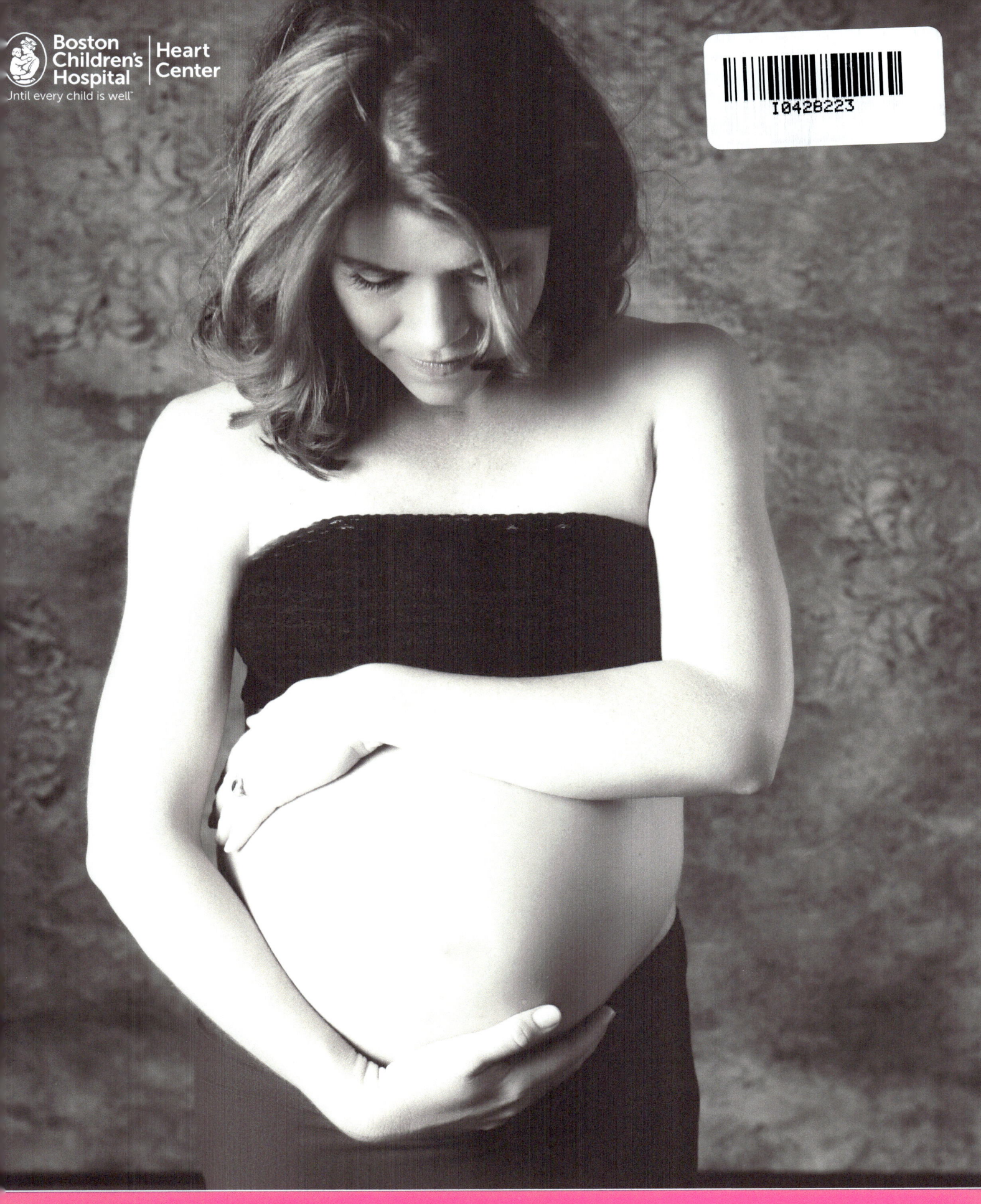

Boston Children's Hospital | Heart Center

Until every child is well™

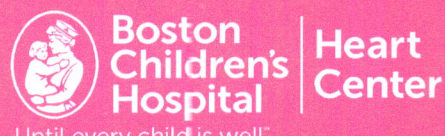

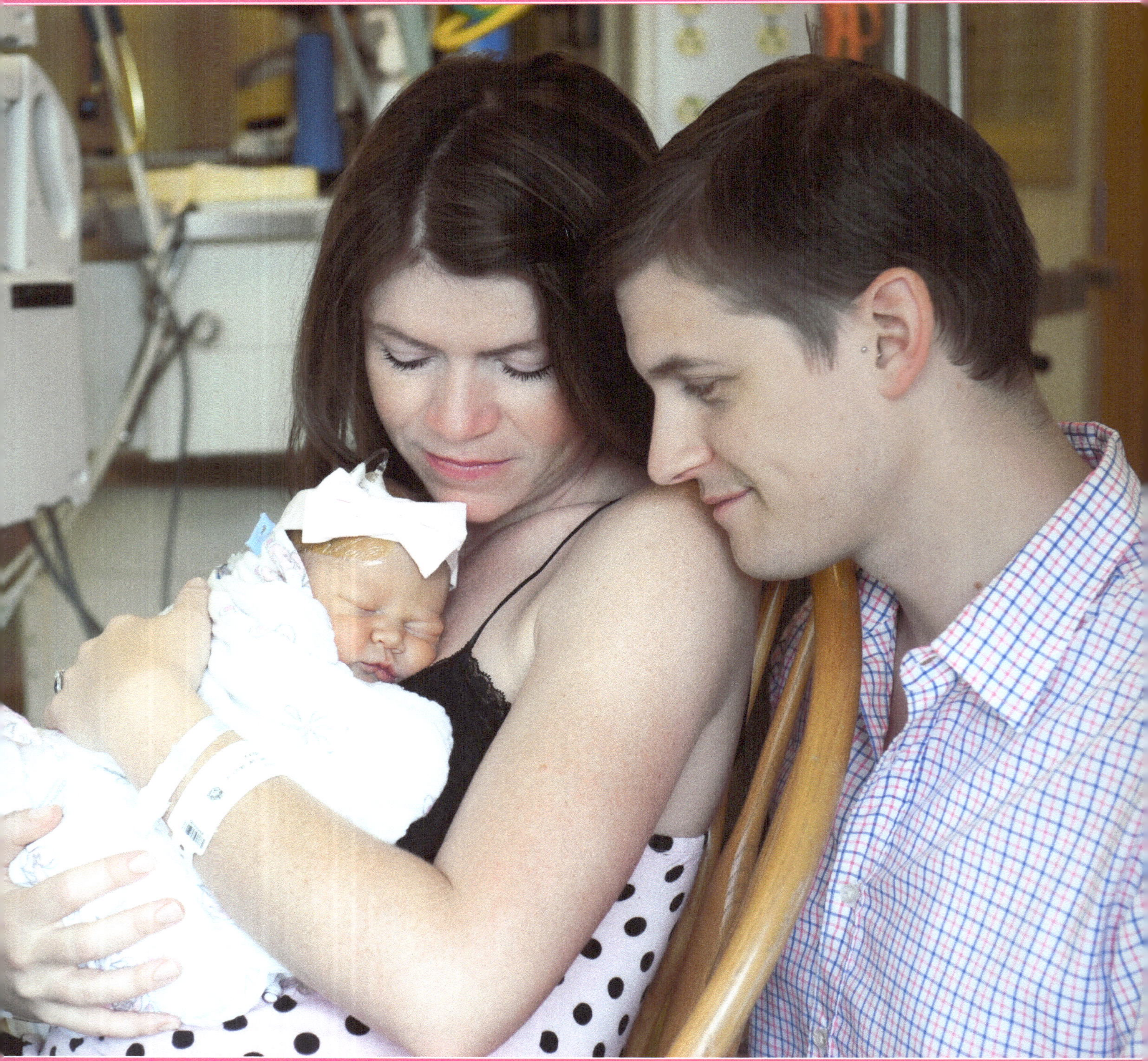

Baby Elliot Grace, enjoying the love and care of her parents in the Cardiac ICU

Boston Children's Hospital Heart Center
300 Longwood Avenue, Farley 2
Boston, MA 02115
617-355-HART
bostonchildrens.org/heart

Boston Children's Hospital Advanced Fetal Care Center
300 Longwood Avenue, Pavilion 2
Boston, MA 02115
617-355-6512
bostonchildrens.org/afcc

An expectant parent's guide to
hypoplastic left heart syndrome and other single ventricle heart defects

Terra Lafranchi, MSN, RN, NP-C

Patricia O'Brien, MSN, RN, CPNP-AC, Michelle Steltzer, MSN, RN, CPNP-AC/PC,

Terry Saia, DNP, APRN, CPNP, Catherine K. Allan, MD, Kimberly H. Barbas, BSN, RN, IBCLC,

Elizabeth D. Blume, MD, Nancy Braudis, RN, MS, CPNP, Roger Breitbart, MD,

David W. Brown, MD, Samantha Butler, PhD, Sitaram Emani, MD, Kevin Friedman, MD,

Jenifer Lightdale, MD, Audrey Marshall, MD, Donna Morash, RN, Diego Porras, MD,

Andrew J. Powell, MD, Rahul Rathod, MD, Amy E. Roberts, MD, Michael N. Singh, MD,

Laurie Oliver Taylor, LICSW, Wayne Tworetzky, MD

This book is dedicated to our incredible heart families for all they have taught us along their unique journeys and for allowing us to share this knowledge with others. Thank you m&m for sharing my love and time so that the dream of this book could become a reality. ~T.L.

Dear Parent,

As a result of key advances in prenatal care and imaging, we can now detect many heart problems during pregnancy. When families first learn about a diagnosis of hypoplastic left heart syndrome (HLHS) or other single ventricle heart defects, they often feel very overwhelmed. At Boston Children's Hospital, we have many years of experience helping children with these conditions and working closely with their parents and other family members since William Norwood, MD, and the cardiac care team at Boston Children's performed the first Norwood surgery for HLHS in 1983.

To better prepare families to care for a child with single ventricle heart disease, we developed this guide to help you navigate the road ahead. Ten families and many clinicians participated in helping to write this book. We know that every child is different, and each journey will be filled with its own unique challenges and celebrations. No matter what your particular path is, your team will be by your side every step of the way.

We hope that this guide will be a resource to refer to, share with others, bring to future fetal cardiology visits and keep with you throughout your baby's first hospital stay.

On behalf of the entire Advanced Fetal Care Center and Fetal Cardiology Program staff,

Terra Lafranchi, MSN, RN, NP-C
Fetal Cardiology Coordinator
terra.lafranchi@cardio.chboston.org

Wayne Tworetzky, MD
Director of Fetal Cardiology
wayne.tworetzky@cardio.chboston.org

Kevin Friedman, MD
Assistant Director of Fetal Cardiology
kevin.friedman@cardio.chboston.org

"Unfortunately, no one ever prepares for a sick baby. The day we learned of Sam's heart, our whole world was turned upside down. All those nagging worries, endless questions and doubt start to creep in. It is a constant refocusing on the positive, finding the tiniest of blessings in every challenge faced along the way with CHD. Sam is now 5 years old and three years after Fontan procedure. For the most part, he's doing wonderfully. It has not been without its challenges but seeing him thrive and live the life I once thought not possible makes even the lowest of lows worth every minute. Sam is the bravest boy with the biggest heart—his love for life inspires me." Sam's parent

---

Information Purposes Only – No Medical Advice

An expectant parent's guide to hypoplastic left heart syndrome and other single ventricle heart defects is offered for information purposes only and is not meant as a substitute for independent medical judgment or the advice of a qualified physician or healthcare professional. *An expectant parent's guide to hypoplastic left heart syndrome* and other single ventricle heart defects is not intended to provide medical advice or clinical services to patients, to verify or approve medical information or credentials, or to make any medical referrals. *An expectant parent's guide to hypoplastic left heart syndrome and other single ventricle heart defects* does not provide professional or medical advice or recommend any particular medical device or service, including recommendations or endorsements through *An expectant parent's guide to hypoplastic left heart syndrome and other single ventricle heart defects*. Users who choose to use information or recommendations made available by the *An expectant parent's guide to hypoplastic left heart syndrome and other single ventricle heart defects* do so at their own risk and should not rely on that information as professional medical advice or use it to replace any relationship with their physicians or other qualified healthcare professionals.

Photography credits:
Spector Photography: p. 1, 2, 14, 59

CONTENTS

INTRODUCTION

Your First Visit to the Advanced Fetal Care Center and Fetal Cardiology Program

During your first visit to the Boston Children's Hospital Advanced Fetal Care Center (AFCC) and Fetal Cardiology Program, you will have a fetal echocardiogram performed. This is a painless, non-invasive test for you that does not affect your baby. It is an ultrasound that gives clear and detailed images of your baby's heart and should take approximately one hour.

Next, you will meet with a pediatric cardiologist (a doctor specially trained in caring for children with heart defects) and a fetal cardiology nurse practitioner (a nurse with advanced training). They will describe how a normal heart looks and works, then review your baby's particular heart condition with you. Our team will talk about the options for medical and surgical treatment, as well as the expected short-term and long-term results of those interventions.

Learning about your baby's heart condition will be an ongoing process that continues after your first visit. We will be ready for any and all questions that you and your family may have after your appointment. Most often, our team will see you again for another echocardiogram and counseling session before your baby is born.

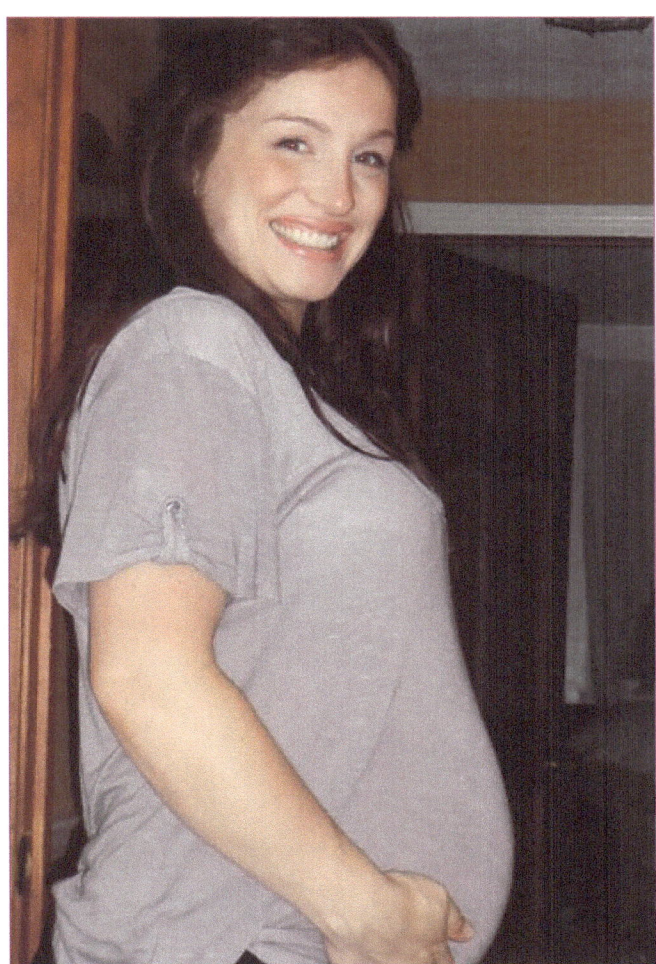

Natalie, pregnant with Mila, a child with a hypoplastic right ventricle

THE DELIVERY AND TIME BEFORE SURGERY

Where will I deliver my baby?

Once your (unborn) baby is found to have a single ventricle heart defect, you should be cared for by a high-risk obstetrician (also called a maternal-fetal medicine, or MFM, doctor) because of your baby's heart problem.

At birth, your baby will need specialized care in the Boston Children's Hospital Cardiac Intensive Care Unit (CICU). For this reason, we recommend that you deliver at an obstetric hospital that is close to Boston Children's. This will allow for a smooth and timely transfer of your baby to our CICU.

Will I need to deliver by C-section?

In most cases, mothers of babies with single ventricle heart defects can give birth vaginally. However, you and your high-risk obstetrician will determine the best mode of delivery.

Will I need a planned delivery?

A planned delivery (induction of labor) may happen at about the 39th week of pregnancy. If you are traveling a long distance for delivery, we may suggest relocating to Boston when you are about 36 to 37 weeks pregnant. Your high-risk obstetrician will make a delivery plan with you based upon your individual health and family needs.

We will be in close communication with your high-risk obstetrician about your delivery plan, and our team will be ready to care for your baby—no matter what the day of the week or time of day that you deliver.

What will happen at the time of delivery?

1. Care in the NICU

The Neonatal Intensive Care Unit (NICU) team will be there at the delivery to help stabilize your baby. Usually babies born with **prenatally diagnosed** HLHS are stable and well-appearing after birth. If your baby is stable, you should have the chance to hold and kiss your baby for a few minutes before your baby is brought to the NICU. A medicine called prostaglandin (PGE1) may be given to your baby through an intravenous (IV) line to keep his or her ductus arteriosus from closing and keep your baby stable before surgery.

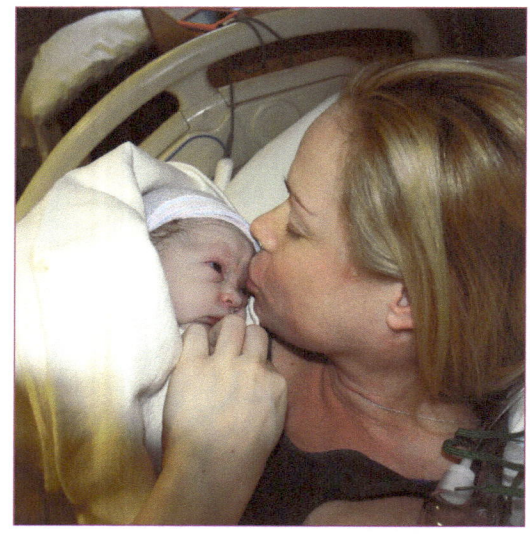

Erin, first kiss to baby Kane in the delivery room

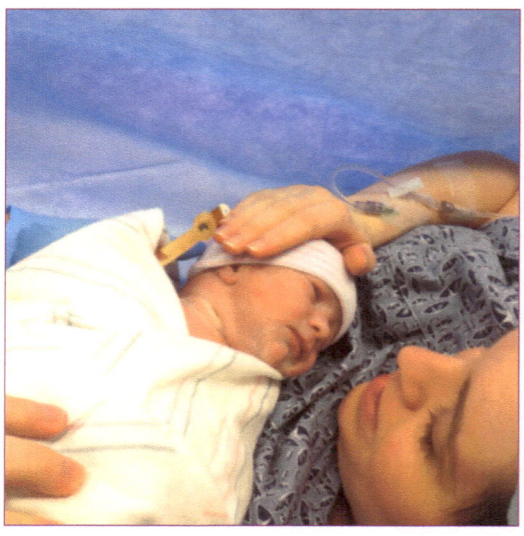

Caitlyn, welcoming baby Genevieve after c-section delivery

The baby will soon be transferred to the CICU at Boston Children's. We will arrange a tour of our CICU before delivery. You will be allowed to come visit your baby as soon as your OB team says you are ready (hopefully within a few hours). Your partner can choose to stay with you or to accompany the baby to the NICU or the CICU.

Occasionally, if your baby is doing well, he or she might stay one or two days in the NICU where you deliver. Even when your baby is in the NICU, he/she is monitored closely by our cardiology team.

2. Care in the CICU

Once your baby comes to the Cardiac Intensive Care Unit (CICU), a team of doctors and nurses will oversee his or her care and confirm the official cardiac diagnosis with an echocardiogram. Your baby might need other diagnostic tests and procedures, such as a cardiac catheterization or cardiac magnetic resonance imaging (MRI) scan, before having surgery.

The CICU doctors will be the main caregivers for your baby while in the CICU, and will work closely with your baby's cardiologist and surgeon to make decisions about the need for more testing and the timing of surgery.

3. Interacting with your baby before surgery

While your baby's surgical plan is being finalized, you will be able to visit at any time. Though your baby will be attached to a heart monitor, and may have a breathing tube, you may still be able to hold and cuddle your baby as much as possible before surgery.

If your baby is stable and the team feels it is safe, your baby may be able to start feeding before surgery. Some babies may not be able to eat by mouth before surgery because of potential risks of intestinal injury before the first operation. If that is the case, nutrition will be given through an IV.

You can pump breast milk which will be stored until your baby is ready to start feeding. Talk about the possibility of "skin to skin" bonding as well as breastfeeding your baby before surgery with your cardiology team and the lactation consultants.

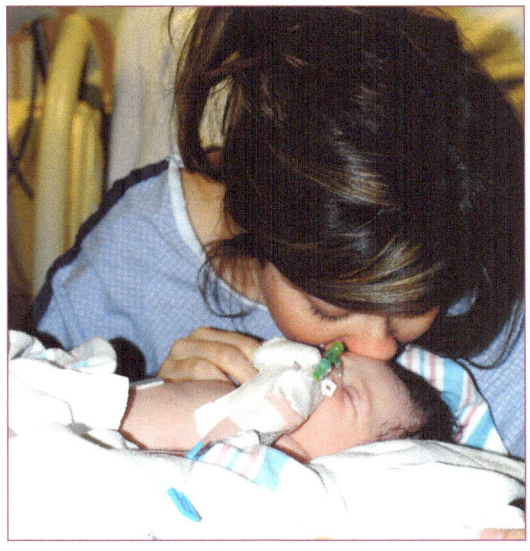
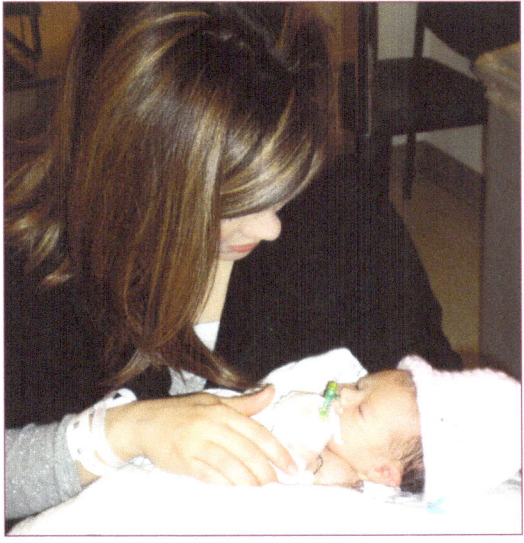

Amber, loving and snuggling baby Addie before Stage 1 operation

4. Special cases

Some babies will need to have a procedure in the cardiac catheterization lab to open the atrial septum (the wall of tissue between the left and right atria).

In rare cases, a baby may become critically ill either at delivery or shortly after, and may need life support. The heart-lung bypass machine (also known as cardiac ECMO, extracorpeal membrane oxygenation), circulates oxygen-rich blood throughout the body. This therapy is immediately available in the CICU for any baby either before or after surgery.

Most babies with single ventricle defects do not need any extra procedures before their operations.

When will the first surgery take place?

You should expect the first surgery to take place within your baby's first week of life, often within the first few days. You will talk about the specific surgical plan in detail with your baby's cardiac surgeon, cardiologist, cardiac intensive care doctor and other team members.

Who will perform my baby's first heart surgery?

A neonatal heart surgeon with special expertise in caring for newborns with complex CHD is always available in our program.

Each week, one of the surgeons is assigned a more flexible schedule so they are available to perform operations for newborns within days of birth.

You will meet your baby's cardiac surgeon and have the opportunity to ask questions shortly after birth and before the operation.

"Mila was put on ECMO five days after her birth after she mysteriously took a bad turn. She was on it for two days. It was terrifying, shocking, humbling, too much to comprehend. What helped was the staff, what always helps is the staff at Boston Children's. There was an ECMO specialist with Mila 24/7; that person never left her side, which was SO comforting! It is hard to look at your child in this state, rather blue, puffy, with a million needles, IV and, the library of drugs being fed into this little body...it's very hard to see AND very hard to even grasp that you are living it. This baby is teaching you more in a week's worth of life than all of your years combined." Mila's parent

---

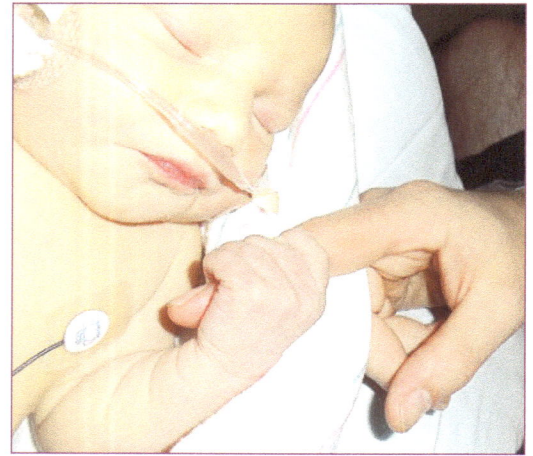

Baby Mila, holding her parent's finger tightly before the Stage 1 operation

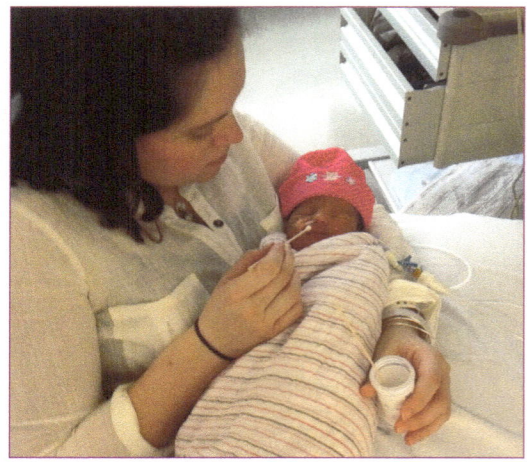

Caitlyn, giving her baby Genevieve pumped colostrum before the Stage 1 operation

Can I donate blood for my baby's surgery?

Blood transfusion is necessary for most types of Stage I treatments. Blood transfused at BCH is largely collected in our own blood donor center, from generous healthy volunteer donors from the general public, many of whom have been donating for years. Each time they donate, they go through a thorough screening process, answering many questions about their medical history and exposure to diseases and behaviors. In addition, the blood is rigorously tested for a wide variety of infectious diseases. Our products are highly regulated; our blood bank is regularly inspected by federal and national agencies; and we are confident that we deliver the safest products available to our patients.

Nevertheless, some families believe that it would be even safer if their loved one received blood donated by the family or a person recruited by the family. This approach —called "directed donation"—was popular when testing was less rigorous, and before it became clear that directed donation offered no advantage over the traditional "volunteer donation" process. Because our goal is to provide the safest blood available for our patients, Boston Children's does not offer directed donations. If you would like more information, you can call the blood donor center at 617-355-6677 or visit halfpints. childrenshospital.org

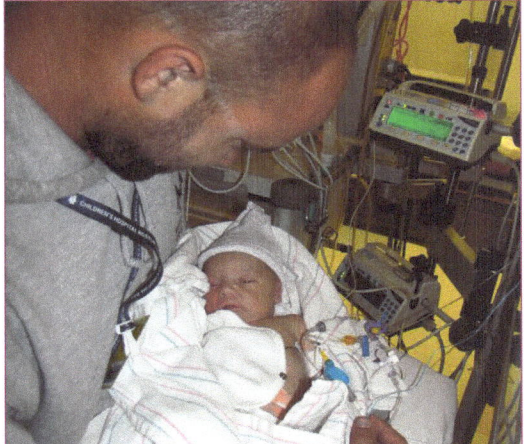

Bill, proudly holding baby Lucas before the Stage 1 operation

Can I have my baby boy circumcised at the time of surgery?

Many parents wonder if their new son can be circumcised during the first surgery or during other cardiac procedures (e.g., catheterization). Due to risks such as infection and bleeding, circumcision is not performed at the time of cardiac surgery. Beyond the first days of life, circumcision becomes a surgical procedure performed by a urologist, and some form of anesthesia is given. Surgeons suggest doing the day surgery procedure between 6-12 months of age. As a rule, we wait until after the Stage 2 surgery so that the baby's circulation is more stable. You may want to ask for a urology consult when your baby is in the hospital for the second surgery to talk about a plan.

Can I have my baby baptized before surgery?

After birth you can ask for your baby to be baptized. Hospital chaplains from all faith backgrounds are on hand for added support. There is also a chapel in the hospital where you can attend services or spend quiet time. Please call 617-355-6664 for more information.

THE NORMAL HEART

The heart is an amazing pump. Its job is to pump blood throughout the body to carry oxygen and nutrients to all of the cells and organs.

Throughout your baby's care, you may hear and read a lot about "red" (oxygen-rich) blood and "blue"(oxygen-poor) blood. These terms aren't meant to describe the actual color of the blood (all blood looks red when it comes out of the body), but they can help you picture the difference between blood that is full of oxygen and blood that is lacking in oxygen. The heart and lungs provide "red" blood to the body.

After the body takes the oxygen it needs from the blood, the oxygen-poor (blue) blood returns to the heart. In the heart, it is collected in the right atrium (right upper collecting chamber), passes through the

tricuspid valve (controls blood flow like a door), enters the right ventricle (right lower pumping chamber, sometimes called "lung pump") and is pumped through the pulmonary valve and pulmonary artery (the large artery that brings blood from the heart to the lungs) into the lungs to pick up oxygen.

Then the oxygen-rich (red) blood leaves the lungs through the pulmonary veins. When it returns to the heart, it is collected in the left atrium (left upper collecting chamber), passes through the mitral valve (controls blood flow like a door), enters the left ventricle (left lower pumping chamber, sometimes called "body pump") and is pumped through the aortic valve and aorta (the large artery that brings blood from the heart to the body) and carries red blood to the body.

Normal Heart

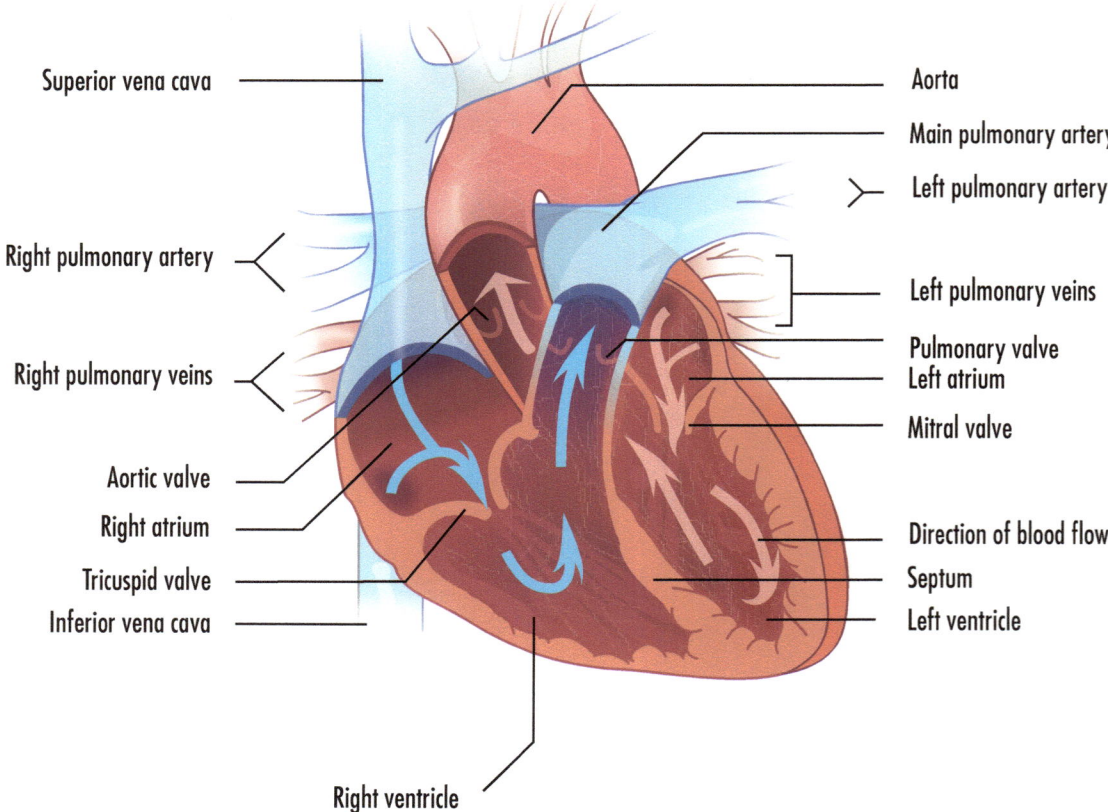

Superior vena cava

Right pulmonary artery

Right pulmonary veins

Aortic valve

Right atrium

Tricuspid valve

Inferior vena cava

Right ventricle

Aorta

Main pulmonary artery

Left pulmonary artery

Left pulmonary veins

Pulmonary valve

Left atrium

Mitral valve

Direction of blood flow

Septum

Left ventricle

HYPOPLASTIC LEFT HEART SYNDROME (HLHS)

In a normal heart, there are two pumping chambers called the right and left ventricle. The right ventricle (sometimes called the lung pump) pumps blue blood to the lungs to pick up oxygen. The left ventricle (sometimes called the body pump) pumps oxygenated red blood to the body. In the fetus, if structures on the left side of the heart are too small, there may be less blood flow to the left ventricle, which prevents the left ventricle from developing normally. The heart will then only have one pumping chamber: the right ventricle. The structures on the left side of the heart that may be too small, or hypoplastic (to varying degrees) may include:

» the **mitral valve** which controls blood flow between the left atrium and left ventricle

» the **left ventricle** which pumps red blood from the heart to the body

» the **aortic valve** which controls blood flow from the left ventricle into the aorta

» the **aorta** which is the large artery that brings red blood from the heart to the body

This defect may be accompanied by other heart defects. There may also be abnormalities in other organs that doctors might not be able to see before the baby is born.

Despite the severity of the condition, a fetus or newborn with HLHS is able to survive because of two connections that allow the blood to be diverted around the small left side of the heart.

Hypoplastic left heart syndrome (HLHS)

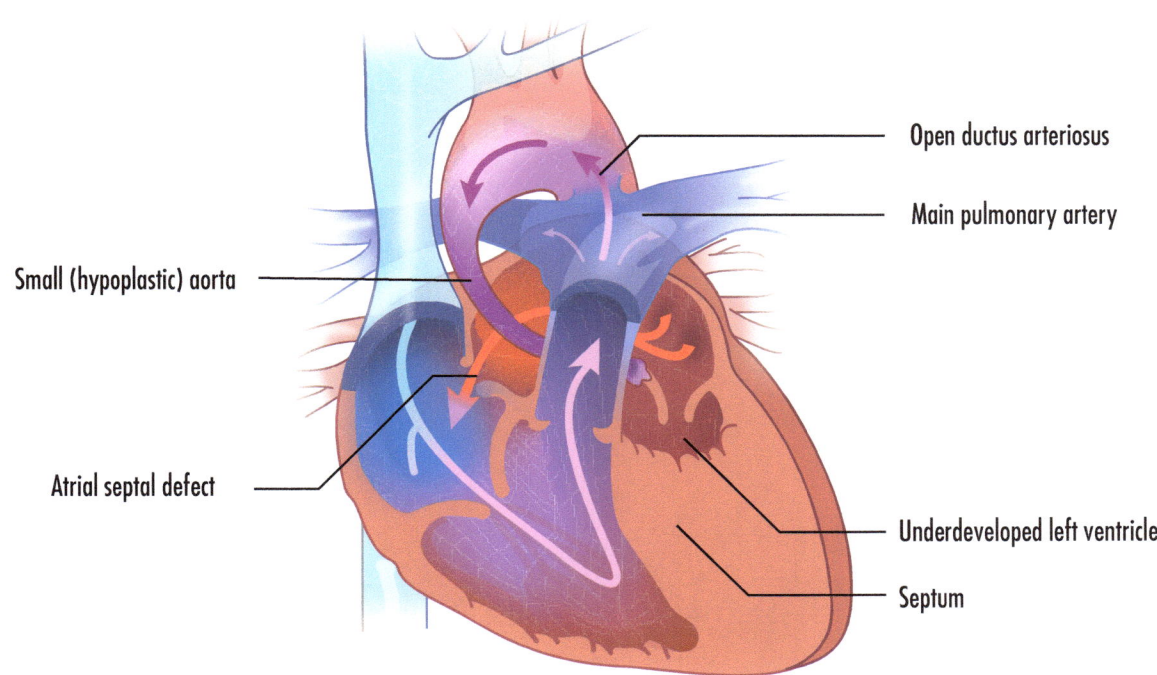

Small (hypoplastic) aorta

Atrial septal defect

Open ductus arteriosus

Main pulmonary artery

Underdeveloped left ventricle

Septum

Patent Ductus Arteriosus (PDA)

The ductus arteriosus is a blood vessel that connects the heart's two biggest arteries (the aorta and the pulmonary artery). Most often it stays open until shortly after birth; In HLHS, as long as the ductus stays open, blood can pass from the right ventricle to the body, letting some oxygen-rich blood circulate.

Patent Foramen Ovale (PFO)

The foramen ovale is a small opening between the right and left atria that is normally present while a fetus is in the womb. It most often closes shortly after birth, but when a baby has HLHS, it's important that the foramen ovale stay open (patent), as this lets blood coming back from the lungs cross from the left atrium to the right atrium and pump to the body through the right ventricle and pulmonary artery.

Most babies will be given a medicine called prostaglandin (PGE1) that works to keep the ductus arteriosus open. This is critical because if the PDA closes, a baby can become very sick due to not enough blood supplying the body. PGE1 is given to the baby through an intravenous line (IV) at birth and the baby will often stay on the medicine until the first surgery or procedure.

Treatment for HLHS

It is not possible to cure HLHS. However, with advances in care, the outlook for babies born with HLHS has improved. Treatment options include: staged surgical procedures; heart transplant; and "comfort care measures" with no heart surgery. The only two options for long-term survival are surgery in the first week of life or heart transplant.

In most cases, the first stage surgery is preferred instead of transplant because the wait for an infant heart can be very long due to a shortage of infant donor hearts. Regrettably, some babies may not survive the wait. In addition, outcomes for the first surgery have significantly improved since Dr. Norwood performed the first operation in the early 1980s. Now we expect many children with HLHS to attend school, take part in many normal childhood activities and grow to adulthood.

The group of infants successfully treated in the 1980s is just reaching their adult years now. The specific options for treatment for your baby's specific heart problem will be discussed with you.

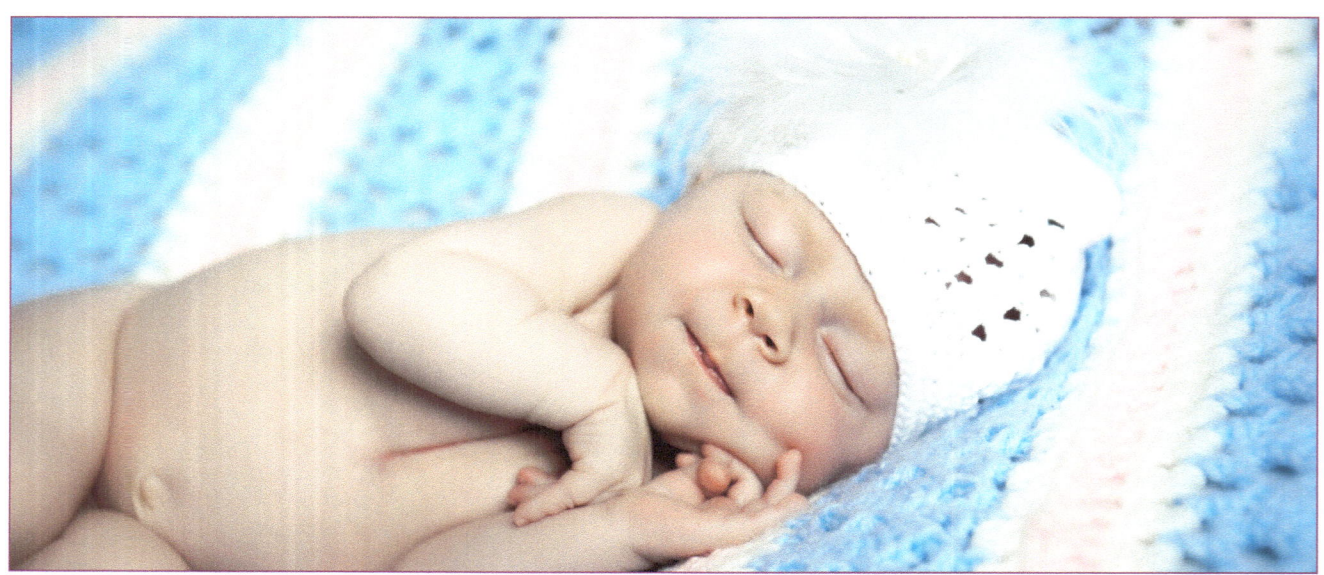

Baby Elliot Grace, recovering from Stage 1 operation

"This photo was taken 3 months after Addie's Fontan surgery. It was on that day at the beach that Tyler and I both realized that everything was okay. Addie was running and laughing and just... well... bursting with joy. There were no indications of surgery or struggle. No one on that beach would have known all that we had been through as a family. She was so happy and so active, giggling and kicking at the tidal pools. Tyler and I didn't say a word to each other. We just watched her in amazement. Tyler took picture after picture and I started tearing up. Finally we both took our attention off of her just long enough to acknowledge that somehow suddenly, everything seemed different. We have the picture hanging in our hallway. I can't look at it without thinking of how blessed we are and how on that day, for the first time in over 2 years, I let out a long sigh of relief." Addie's parent

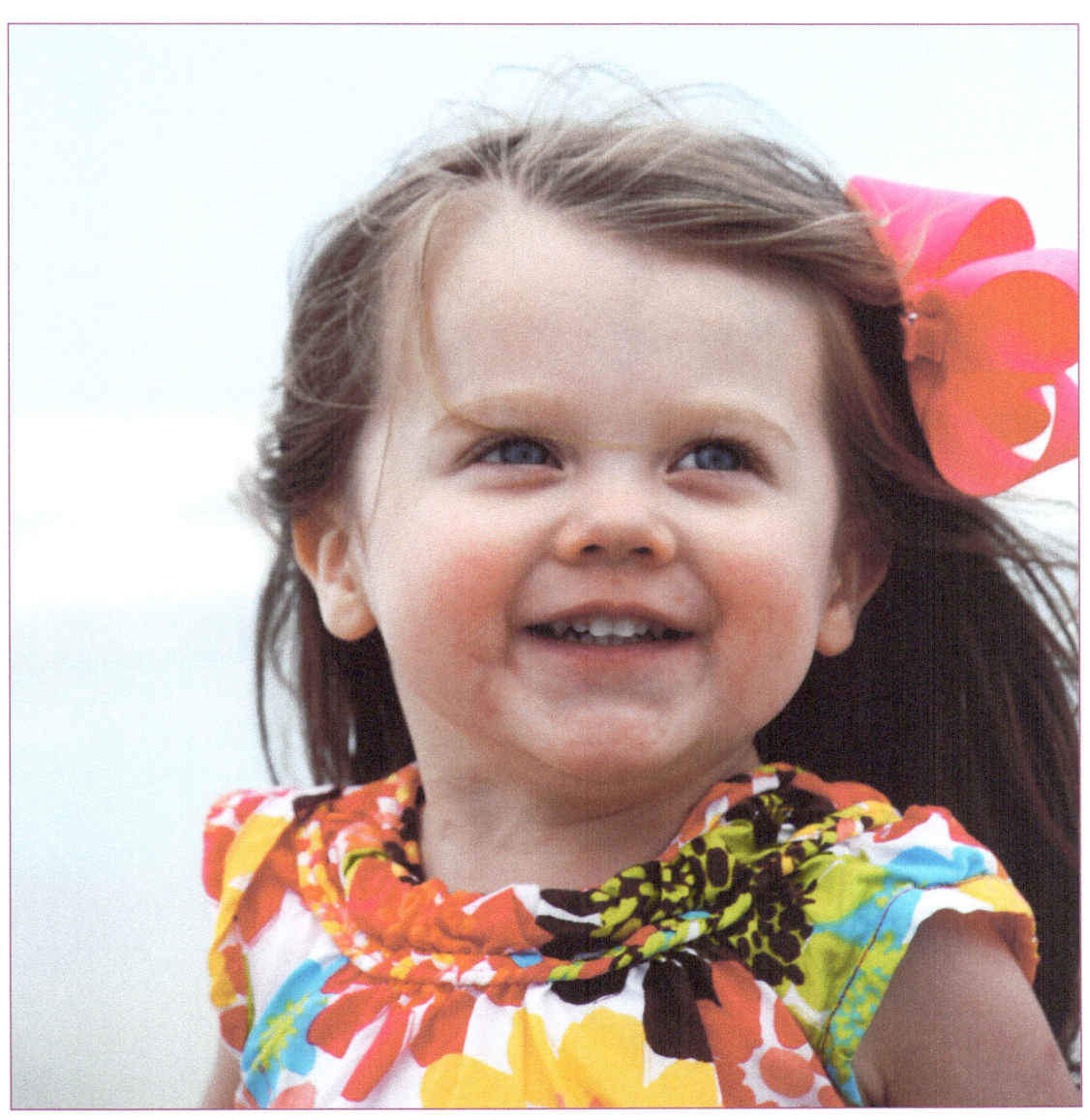

Addie, on the beach after Fontan operation

OTHER SINGLE VENTRICLE HEART DEFECTS

"Single ventricle heart defect" is a term used to describe several very different congenital heart defects that share the same basic problem: one ventricle did not grow normally and is not able to pump blood adequately. The hypoplastic ventricle could be the right ventricle (designed to pump blood to the lungs) or the left ventricle (designed to pump blood to the body). There may also be abnormalities in other organs that doctors may or may not be able to see before the baby is born.

Below is a list of single ventricle heart defects and a brief definition. The list is provided in two categories: 1) Hypoplastic Left Ventricle (or Single Right Ventricle) and 2) Hypoplastic Right Ventricle (or Single Left Ventricle).

Your baby may have one of the single ventricle heart defects listed below or your baby may have a variation or combination of different heart defects. Your cardiologist will tell you in detail the exact type of single ventricle heart defect your baby has and the expected prognosis and treatment choices.

Hypoplastic Left Ventricle Defects (or Single Right Ventricle)

Hypoplastic Left Heart Syndrome (HLHS)
(see previous section, page 13)

Mitral Valve Atresia (MA)
» In a normal heart, there is a mitral valve between the left atrium and left ventricle of the heart. This valve acts as a doorway between the two chambers and controls blood flow between the chambers.

» In this defect, the mitral valve did not develop correctly and blood can't flow from the left atrium into the left ventricle, preventing the left ventricle from developing normally. The left ventricle then becomes too small to pump blood to the body as designed. This defect might be combined with other heart defects.

Double Outlet Right Ventricle (DORV) and Hypoplastic Left Ventricle
» In a normal heart, the pulmonary artery is connected to the right ventricle to bring blood to the lungs to pick up oxygen, and the aorta is connected to the left ventricle.

» In this defect, the pulmonary artery and the aorta are both connected to the right ventricle instead of just the pulmonary artery. In some cases, this stops the left ventricle from growing normally. The left ventricle then becomes too small to pump blood to the body as designed. This defect might be combined with other heart defects.

Double Inlet Right Ventricle (DIRV)
» In a normal heart the right atrium is connected to the right ventricle and the left atrium is connected to the left ventricle.

» In this defect, both the right and left atria connect to the right ventricle through the tricuspid and mitral valves. In some cases, this keeps the left ventricle from developing normally. The left ventricle then becomes too small to pump blood to the body as designed. This defect might be combined with other heart defects.

Right Dominant Unbalanced Atrioventricular (AV) Canal

» In a normal heart, there is a septum that divides the right and left side of the heart.

» In this defect, there is a hole in the septum in the center of the heart, where the upper chambers (the atria) and the lower chambers (the ventricles) meet. Instead of two valves (e.g., tricuspid and mitral valves) separating the atria and ventricles, there is only one common AV valve. Also, the septum is not in the center, but off to one side (unbalanced), making the left side of the heart smaller than the right side.

Hypoplastic Right Ventricle Defects (or Single Left Ventricle)

Tricuspid Valve Atresia

» In a normal heart, the tricuspid valve is positioned between the right atrium and right ventricle of the heart. This valve acts as a doorway between the two chambers and controls blood flow between the chambers.

» In this defect, the tricuspid valve does not develop correctly and blood cannot flow from the right atrium into the right ventricle, which stops the right ventricle from developing normally. As a result, the right ventricle is too small to pump blood to the lungs as designed. This defect can be combined with other heart defects.

Pulmonary Atresia with Intact Ventricular Septum (PA/IVS) and Hypoplastic Right Ventricle

» In a normal heart, there is a pulmonary valve that controls blood flow from the right ventricle into the pulmonary artery.

» In this defect, a solid sheet of tissue formed where the pulmonary valve should be, and the valve stays closed. Blood is unable to flow from right ventricle to the lungs to pick up oxygen. In some cases, the right ventricle does not develop as it should and becomes too small to pump blood to the lungs as designed. This defect can be combined with other heart defects

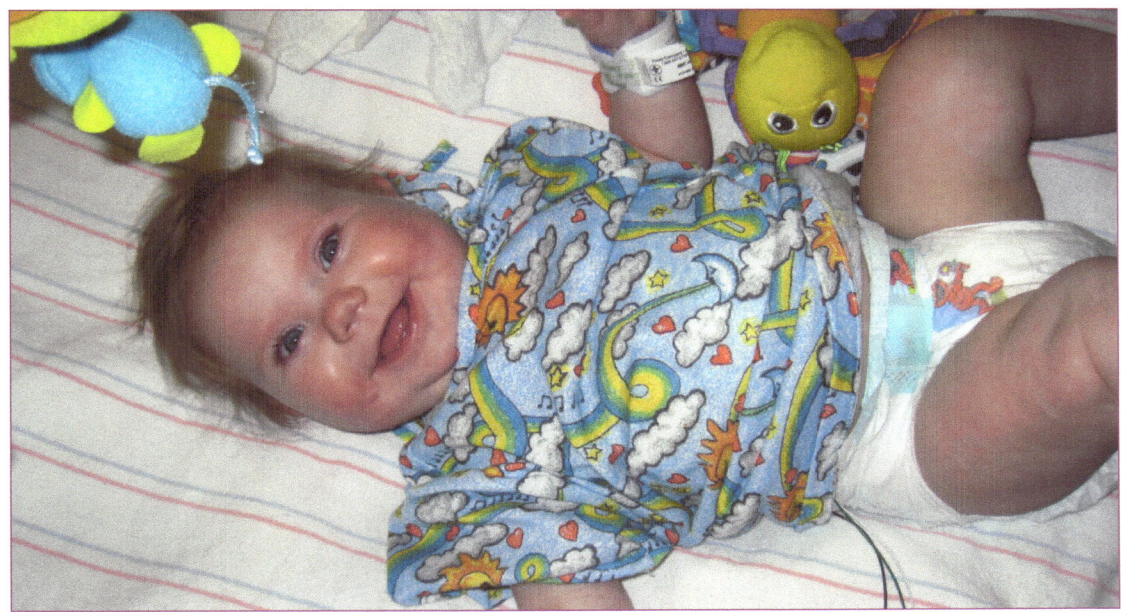

Baby Kaya, on cardiology floor after Glenn operation for hypoplastic right ventricle

Double Inlet Left Ventricle (DILV)

» In a normal heart the right atrium is connected to the right ventricle and the left atrium is connected to the left ventricle.

» In this defect, both the right and left atria connect to the left ventricle. In some cases, this prevents the right ventricle from developing normally. The right ventricle then becomes too small to pump blood to the lungs as designed. This defect can be combined with other heart defects.

Left Dominant Unbalanced AV Canal

» In a normal heart, there is a septum that divides the right and left side of the heart.

» In this defect, there is a hole in the septum in the center of the heart, where the upper chambers (the atria) and the lower chambers (the ventricles) meet. Instead of two valves (e.g., tricuspid and mitral valves) separating the atria and ventricles, there is only one common AV valve. Also, the septum is not in the center, but off to one side (unbalanced) making the right side of the heart smaller than the left side of the heart.

What causes single ventricle heart defects?

There is no clear reason why these congenital heart defects happen. It is thought to be a complex interaction of genetics and the environment.

Some congenital heart defects may be genetic, caused by either a defect in a gene or an abnormality in a chromosome. Your doctor might recommend that you have an amniocentesis—a procedure that removes a sample of fluid from the amniotic sac around the fetus for testing—to screen for any identifiable chromosomal problems during the pregnancy.

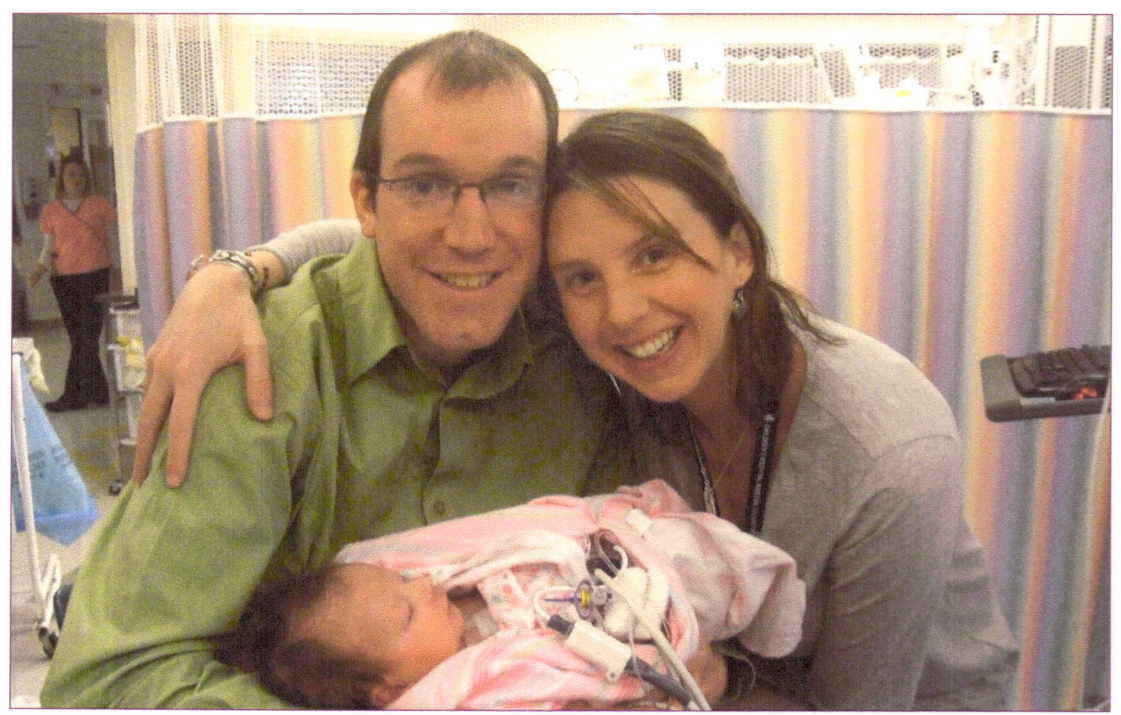

Brian and Molly, holding baby Haven before the Stage 1 operation for PA/IVS with hypoplastic right ventricle

TREATMENTS FOR SINGLE VENTRICLE HEART DEFECTS

It is not possible to cure single ventricle heart defects and create a structurally normal heart. Therefore, in most cases, surgery is palliative (improves the blood flow patterns to improve cardiac symptons). The goal of the surgeries is to support the functioning right or left ventricle to do the work normally done by two ventricles. Most babies with single ventricle heart defects (including HLHS) need a three-stage surgical plan. Your baby will also need cardiac catheterizations and may need future surgeries beyond the third stage operation.

First Stage operation

The first stage operation is most often performed in the first week of life. The goal of the first surgery is to optimize blood flow to the body and the lungs. In babies with a small left ventricle and aorta, blood flow to the aorta and body needs to be established. We will talk with you about the type of first surgery that we think your baby will need.

The next section (Types of First Stage operations for Single Ventricle Heart Defects) will give more information about these surgeries and their recoveries.

a. **If blood flow to the body is not enough,** below is a list of all Stage 1 procedures:

» Stage 1 Norwood operation with BT Shunt (page 20).

» Stage 1 Norwood operation with Sano Modification (page 21).

» Hybrid Procedure (page 22).

b. **If blood flow to the lungs is not enough,** below are procedures to increase the flow:

» BT Shunt (page 23).

» PDA Stent (page 24).

c. **If blood flow to the lungs is too much,** the pulmonary artery may be surgically made smaller by placing a band to narrow its size (known as a PA Band) to control blood flow. This is uncommon. (Page 23).

d. **If blood flow to the body and lungs is not too much or not too little,** an operation during the newborn period may not be needed and the second stage surgery (bidirectional Glenn Shunt) may be performed at 4 to 8 months of age. This is uncommon and ensuring that the blood flow is balanced can require close monitoring.

Second Stage operation (bidirectional Glenn shunt)

The second stage operation is most often performed between 4 and 6 months of age, or sometimes earlier based on your baby's unique needs (Page 26).

Third Stage operation (Fontan)

The third stage operation is most often performed between 18 months and 4 years (page 28). The Fontan circulation (blood flow) will:

» separate the oxygen-deprived blue blood from the red blood within the heart

» allow the single, normal-sized ventricle to pump oxygen-rich red blood to the rest of the body

» allow blood to flow passively to the lungs (does not need a pump)

We expect that your baby will need these three surgeries (this plan may change):

1) _____

2) _____

3) _____

TYPES OF **FIRST STAGE OPERATIONS** FOR SINGLE VENTRICLE HEART DEFECTS

Below is a list of all of the different types of first stage operations. Ask your team what surgery your baby will likely have and review that section below. The type of surgery may change depending on your baby's unique heart anatomy, weight, and surgeon preference.

The first stage operation for a single ventricle heart defect is usually performed during the first week of life, often within the first few days after birth.

The expected hospital stay is approximately one or two months after birth. This time frame can vary based on your baby's specific circumstances and could be longer or shorter, or in rare instances, until the second surgery.

Babies typically have oxygen saturation levels between 75% and 85% after first stage operations, but each patient is unique. This is an easily obtained assesment of how your baby is doing.

STAGE 1 Norwood operation with Modified Blalock-Taussig Shunt (BT Shunt)

The primary goal of the Norwood operation is to rebuild the aorta and bring blood to the rest of the body. The membrane separating the right and left atrial chambers

(atrial septum) is also removed. Because the pulmonary artery is used in the reconstruction of the aorta, the surgery must provide another way for blood to get to the lungs. The BT Shunt is one way to do this. In this portion of the operation, a GORE-TEX® tube graft is used to divert some blood from a large blood vessel off the aorta directly to the pulmonary artery (the blood vessel going to the lungs).

Recovery: After the Stage 1 Norwood with BT shunt your baby will go back to the CICU while still under anesthesia (this is also called being sedated) and on a breathing machine (ventilator). Your baby will have many tubes, wires and equipment to monitor all of their body systems in the first days after surgery. The first 48 hours after surgery are vital, and doctors and nurses will be making frequent adjustments to your baby's medicines and to the breathing machine (ventilator) during this time. It's very important that a newborn's growing lungs are healthy and get a strong and steady flow of blood. If babies have sick lungs, it can affect how they will recover from surgery and if they will have other issues. Your baby's heart rhythm will be watched closely and will be treated if not normal. You may see lots of activity at your baby's bedside during the first night after surgery in particular. This is expected, and

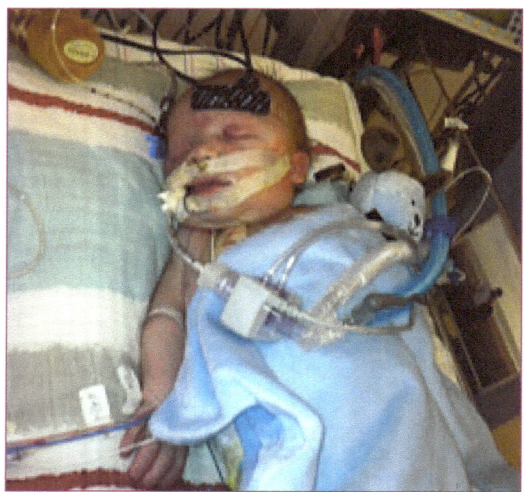

Baby Finn, in CICU after Stage 1 operation

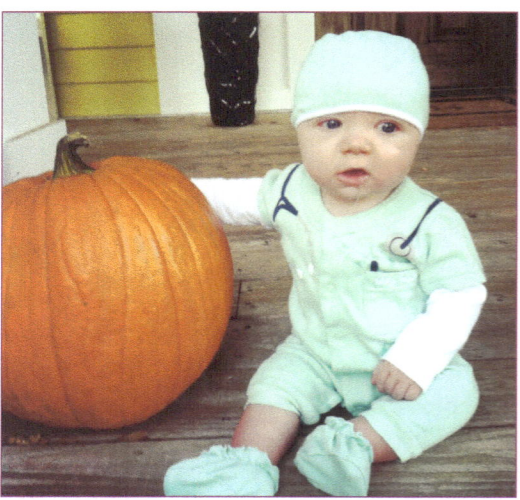

Baby Finn, one month after Glenn operation

the doctors and nurses in the CICU will keep you closely informed of your baby's progress.

Many babies will have a delayed sternal closure: for a few days after surgery the breastbone and skin are left partly open but with a protective covering. Because soft tissue and even heart muscle can become swollen after surgery, leaving the incision partly open gives time for the swelling to go down before the incision is closed. Your baby's surgeon will close the incision fully at the bedside a few days after surgery.

Babies will usually stay sedated until the incision is closed. Once this happens, your baby will be allowed to move more and be more aware of surroundings. They will be given less sedation medicine but will still receive pain medicine. The time that your baby will need to be on a breathing machine could vary from several days to several weeks based on your baby's status and risk factors before surgery. In many cases, your baby will be slowly weaned off the breathing machine several days following surgery. Medicines that support the heart function will be decreased or given by mouth as your baby gets better. Feedings will be started. When your baby is stable and no longer needs the specialized care in the Cardiac Intensive Care Unit, they will be transferred to the cardiology ward to continue their recovery. This is a positive forward step in the recovery process. Please see page 31 for more information about "Preparing to Take Your Baby Home."

STAGE 1 Norwood operation with Sano Modification

The Norwood operation will rebuild the aorta and connect it to the ventricle. This will allow a single pumping chamber to pump blood into the aorta and bring blood to the rest of the body. In order for the blood to flow easily throughout the heart, surgeons also remove the membrane separating the right and left atrial chambers (atrial septum). Because the pulmonary artery is used in the rebuilding of the aorta, pulmonary blood flow must be supplied through an alternate route. In the case of a Sano Modification, a conduit (tube) is used to directly connect the right ventricle to the pulmonary arteries.

Recovery: Following Stage 1 Norwood with Sano Modification your baby will return to the CICU while still under anesthesia (this is also called being sedated) and on a breathing machine (ventilator). Your baby will have many tubes, wires and equipment to monitor all of their body systems in the first days after surgery. The first 48 hours after surgery are vital, and doctors and nurses will be making frequent adjustments to your baby's medicines and to the breathing machine (ventilator) during this time. It's very important that a newborn's growing lungs are healthy and get a strong and steady flow of blood. If babies have sick lungs, it can affect how they will recover from surgery and if they will have other issues. Your baby's heart rhythm will be watched closely and will be treated if not normal. You may see lots of activity at your baby's bedside during the first night after surgery in particular. This is expected, and the doctors and nurses in the CICU will keep you closely informed of your baby's progress.

Many babies will have a delayed sternal closure: for a few days after surgery the breastbone and skin are left partly open but with a protective covering. Because soft tissue and even heart muscle can become swollen after surgery, leaving the incision partly open gives time for the swelling to go down before the incision is closed. Your baby's surgeon will close the incision fully at the bedside several days after surgery.

Babies will usually stay sedated until the incision is closed. Once this happens, your baby will be allowed to move more and be more aware of surroundings. They will be given less sedation medicine but will still receive pain medicine. The time that your baby will need to be on a breathing machine could vary from several days to several weeks based on your baby's status and risk factors before surgery. In many cases, your baby will be slowly weaned off the breathing machine several days following surgery. Medicines that support the heart function will be decreased or given by mouth as your baby gets better. Feedings will be started. When your baby is stable and no longer needs the specialized care in the Cardiac Intensive Care Unit, they will be transferred to the cardiology ward to continue their recovery. This is a positive forward step in the recovery process. Please see page 31 for more information about "Preparing to Take Your Baby Home."

Hybrid Procedure

The Hybrid Procedure is used for some selected or very high-risk babies with a single ventricle defect whose condition is not stable enough for surgery that requires a heart-lung bypass machine. The Hybrid Procedure combines catheterization (insertion of a flexible tube into a heart chamber or vessel) and minimally invasive surgery. Interventional cardiologists insert a stent into the ductus arteriosus (PDA) to keep it open, allowing blood to flow from the single ventricle through this stented PDA to the aorta and around the body. Then surgeons place pulmonary artery bands (PA bands) around the right and left pulmonary artery branches to control the amount of blood going to lungs. For these babies, the second stage surgery will be more complex because the aortic arch repair will be done in addition to the Glenn procedure.

Recovery: After The Hybrid Procedure your baby will go back to the CICU while still under anesthesia (this is also called being sedated) and on a breathing machine (ventilator). Your baby will have many tubes, wires and equipment to monitor all of their body systems in the first days after surgery. The first 48 hours after surgery are vital, and

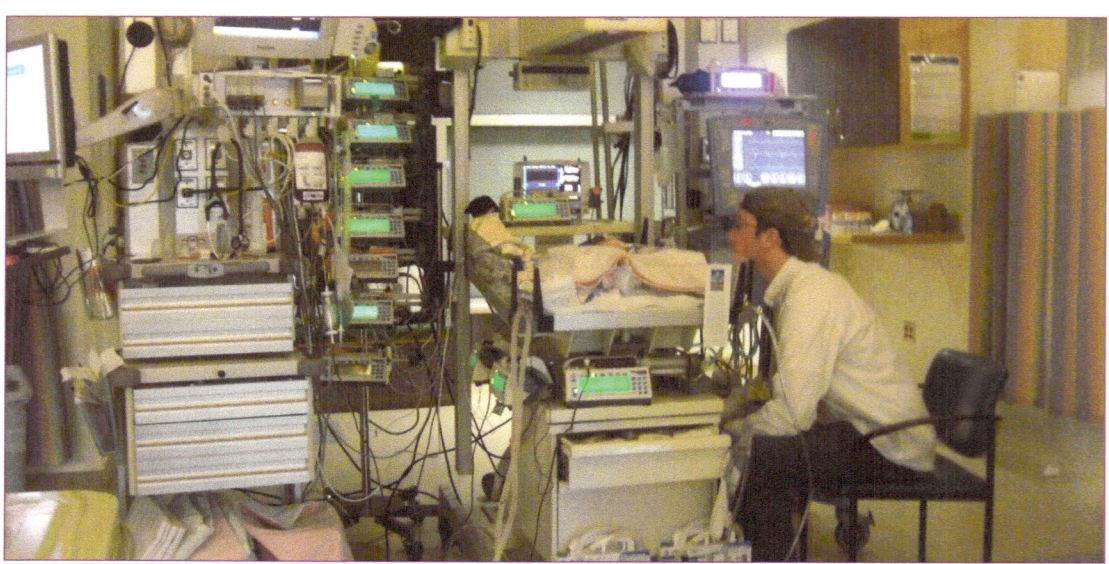

Brian, watching over baby Haven's bedside after Stage 1 operation

doctors and nurses will be making frequent adjustments to your baby's medicines and to the breathing machine (ventilator) during this time. It's very important that a new-born's growing lungs are healthy and get a strong and steady flow of blood. If babies have sick lungs, it can affect how they will get better from surgery and if they will have other issues. Your baby's heart rhythm will be watched closely and will be treated if not normal. You may see lots of activity at your baby's bedside during the first night after surgery in particular. This is expected, and the doctors and nurses in the CICU will keep you closely informed of your baby's progress.

The time that your baby will need to be on a breathing machine could vary from several days to several weeks based on your baby's status and risk factors before surgery. In many cases, the baby will be slowly weaned off the breathing machine several days following surgery. Medicines that support the heart function will be decreased or given by mouth as your baby gets better. Feedings will be started. When your baby is stable and no longer needs the specialized care in the Cardiac Intensive Care Unit, they will be transferred to the cardiology ward to continue their recovery. This is a positive forward step in the recovery process. Please see page 31 for more information about "Preparing to Take Your Baby Home."

Modified Blalock-Taussig Shunt (BT Shunt)

The BT Shunt is used to provide blood flow to the lungs with the placement of a GO-RE-TEX® tube graft that connects a large blood vessel off the aorta to the pulmonary artery (the blood vessel going to the lungs). This operation is used for babies who do not have enough blood flow to the lungs, but have enough blood flow to the body, such as in pulmonary atresia with intact ventricular septum and other problems with small right ventricles.

Recovery: After a BT shunt, your baby will go back to the CICU while still under anesthesia (this is also called being sedated) and on a

breathing machine (ventilator). Your baby will have many tubes, wires and equipment to monitor all of their body systems in the first days after surgery. The first 48 hours after surgery are vital, and doctors and nurses will be making frequent adjustments to your baby's medicines and to the breathing machine during this time. It's very important that a newborn's growing lungs are healthy and get a strong, steady flow of blood. If babies have sick lungs, it can affect how they will get better from surgery and if they will have other issues. Your baby's heart rhythm will be watched closely and will be treated if not normal. You may see lots of activity at your baby's bedside during the first night after surgery in particular. This is expected, and the doctors and nurses in the CICU will keep you closely informed of your baby's progress.

Over the next several days, your baby will be slowly weaned off the breathing machine. Medicines that support the heart function will be decreased or given by mouth as your baby heals. Feedings will be started. When your baby is stable and no longer needs the specialized care in the Cardiac Intensive Care Unit, they will be transferred to the cardiology ward to continue their recovery. This is a positive forward step in the recovery process Please see page 31 for more information about "Preparing to Take Your Baby Home."

Pulmonary Artery Band (PA BAND)

PA Band surgery is needed when there is too much blood flow to the lungs. The surgeon will place a tie around the main pulmonary artery to narrow it and stop too much blood from going to the lungs. This will also help protect the pulmonary vessels. This is the least common operation done for single ventricle defects.

Recovery: After PA Band Surgery, your baby will go back to the CICU while still under anesthesia (this is also called being sedated) and on a breathing machine (ventilator). Your baby will have many tubes, wires and equipment to monitor all of their body systems in the first days after surgery.

The first 48 hours after surgery are vital, and doctors and nurses will be making frequent adjustments to your baby's medicines and to the breathing machine (ventilator) during this time. It's very important that a newborn's growing lungs are healthy and get a strong, steady flow of blood. If babies have sick lungs, it can affect how they will get better from surgery and if they will have other issues. Your baby's heart rhythm will be watched closely and will be treated if not normal. You may see lots of activity at your baby's bedside during the first night after surgery in particular. This is expected, and the doctors and nurses in the CICU will keep you closely informed of your baby's progress.

Over the next several days, your baby will be slowly weaned off the breathing machine. Medicines that support the heart function will be decreased or given by mouth as your baby gets better. Feedings will be started. When your baby is stable and no longer needs the specialized care in the Cardiac Intensive Care Unit, they will be transferred to the cardiology ward to continue their recovery. This is a positive forward step in the recovery process. Please see page 31 for more information about "Preparing to Take Your Baby Home."

Patent Ductus Arteriosus (PDA) Stent

PDA Stent placement is a procedure that is performed in the cath lab, not in the operating room. A flexible tube is placed through a vessel at the top of the leg into the heart. An interventional cardiologist will place a device called a stent into the PDA to keep it open. This allows blood to flow from the single ventricle through the stented PDA to the lungs.

The decision to place a PDA stent is most often made when there are other issues that make the baby more high-risk for a surgical procedure that calls for a heart-lung bypass machine. Your cardiologist will tell you why your baby would benefit from a PDA stent. This is a temporary procedure followed by a surgical procedure later.

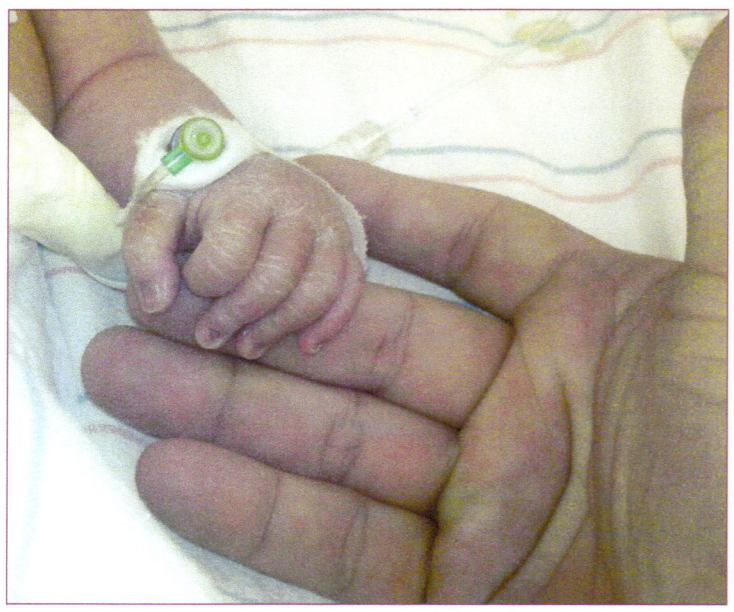

Baby Brooklyn, holding her father's finger after Stage 1 operation

Recovery: After PDA Stent your baby will go back to the CICU while still under anesthesia (this is also called being sedated) and on a breathing machine (ventilator). Your baby will have many tubes, wires and equipment to monitor all of their body systems. The first 48 hours after surgery are vital, and doctors and nurses will be making frequent adjustments to your baby's medicines and to the breathing machine (ventilator) during this time. It's very important that a newborn's growing lungs are healthy and get a strong, steady flow of blood. If babies have sick lungs, it can affect how they will get better from surgery and if they will have other issues. Your baby's heart rhythm will be watched closely and will be treated if not normal. You may see lots of activity at your baby's bedside during the first night after surgery in particular. This is expected, and the doctors and nurses in the CICU will keep you closely informed of your baby's progress.

Over the next several days, your baby should be slowly weaned off the breathing machine. Medicines that support the heart function will be decreased or given by mouth as your baby gets better. Feedings will be started. When your baby is stable and no longer needs the specialized care in the Cardiac Intensive Care Unit, they will be transferred to the cardiology ward to continue their recovery. This is a positive forward step in the recovery process. Please see page 31 for more information about "Preparing to Take Your Baby Home."

"Make sure you listen to the doctors' and nurses' advice and leave the hospital sometimes. The ICU is like a casino where the lights never shut off, the rounds and the checkups never stop. It is easy to go crazy. Get out and take a walk, sleep at home or a hotel. It is absolutely necessary to unwind, decompress, and think about what the day has brought you. Of course, the guilt of walking away from your child is excruciating, but you have to find solace in the fact that your child is being looked after every second by a highly trained nurse in the best children's hospital for cardiac issues in the world. You can leave for a while, you really can." Mila's parent

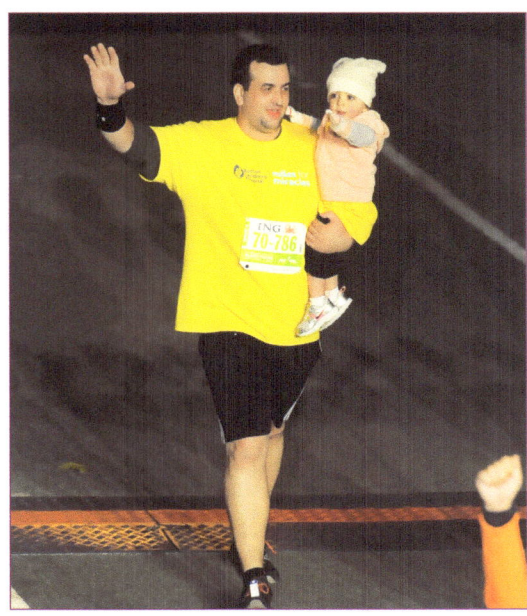

Brooklyn's father carrying her across the marathon finish line after her Glenn operation

SECOND STAGE OPERATION FOR SINGLE VENTRICLE DEFECTS: BIDIRECTIONAL GLENN SHUNT

Your baby will likely need a cardiac catheterization or cardiac MRI before the second stage (bidirectional Glenn) operation and may have to spend the night in the hospital afterwards. The purpose of these imaging studies is to measure the pressures and function of the heart and do interventions if needed. Many patients require catheter-based interventions to improve the Glenn surgery outcomes.

Preparation for the Glenn surgery will include a one-day outpatient pre-operative assessment by our cardiology and cardiac anesthesia team. Your baby's exact plan will be explained in detail to you.

The bidirectional Glenn operation (or superior cavopulmonary anastamosis) guides blood flow from the baby's upper body straight into the lungs by making a connection between the vein carrying blood back to the heart from the head and arms (called the superior vena cava) and the pulmonary artery. This is all natural tissue so it will grow with your baby and is the right size to provide enough pulmonary blood flow.

If a tube (shunt or conduit) to carry blood flow to the lungs was placed during your baby's first operation, it is removed during this procedure. Blue blood from the upper body now flows straight to the lungs without

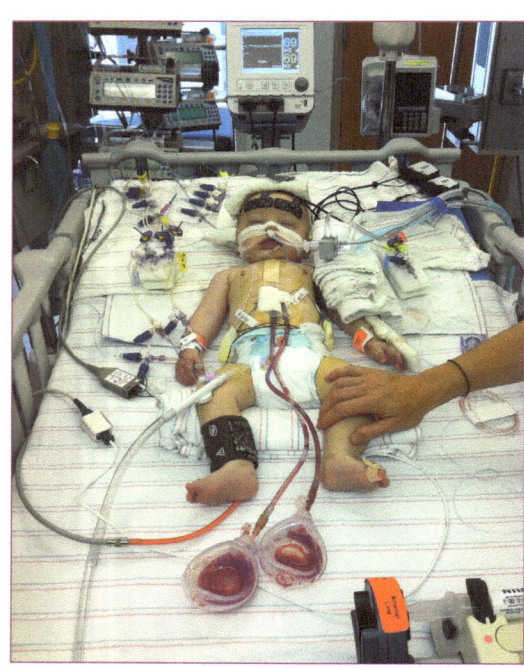

Kane, in CICU after Glenn operation

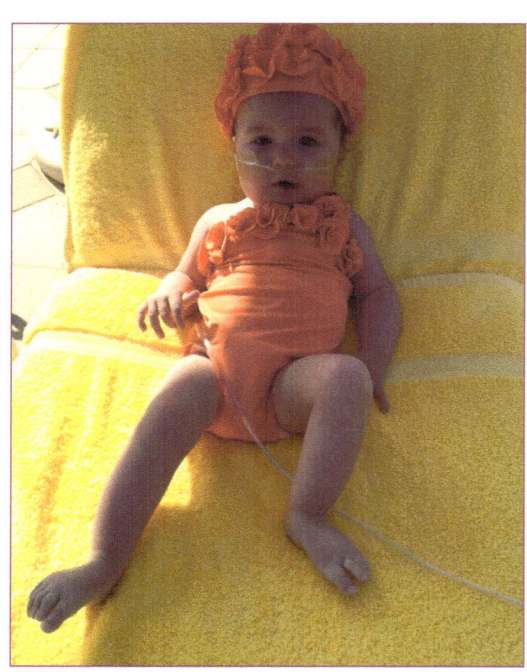

Mary, on vacation after Glenn operation (in rare cases, babies will need oxygen at home)

the help of the ventricle. There is less blood going through the heart so the workload of the heart is less after the surgery. There is still mixing of blue blood returning from the lower body with red blood in the ventricle so the baby's oxygen levels stay in the 80 percent range. The cardiac system is more stable after the surgery and an improvement in growth and development is often seen after the bidirectional Glenn operation.

Average age at time of surgery: 4 to 6 months; timing will depend on the unique needs of your baby.

Expected hospital stay: Seven to ten days. The recovery process after this procedure is usually less complicated than recovery after the first stage. Babies may only need to spend one or two days in the Cardiac Intensive Care Unit, though this will vary based on the needs of the individual child. Higher superior vena cava pressure may happen resulting in temporary swelling of the face, neck or arms. This can also result in a "Glenn headache." Medicines and elevating the baby's head may help relieve the increased pressures.

Oxygen saturation levels: Babies usually have oxygen saturation levels of 80 percent after this surgery, but each patient's situation is unique.

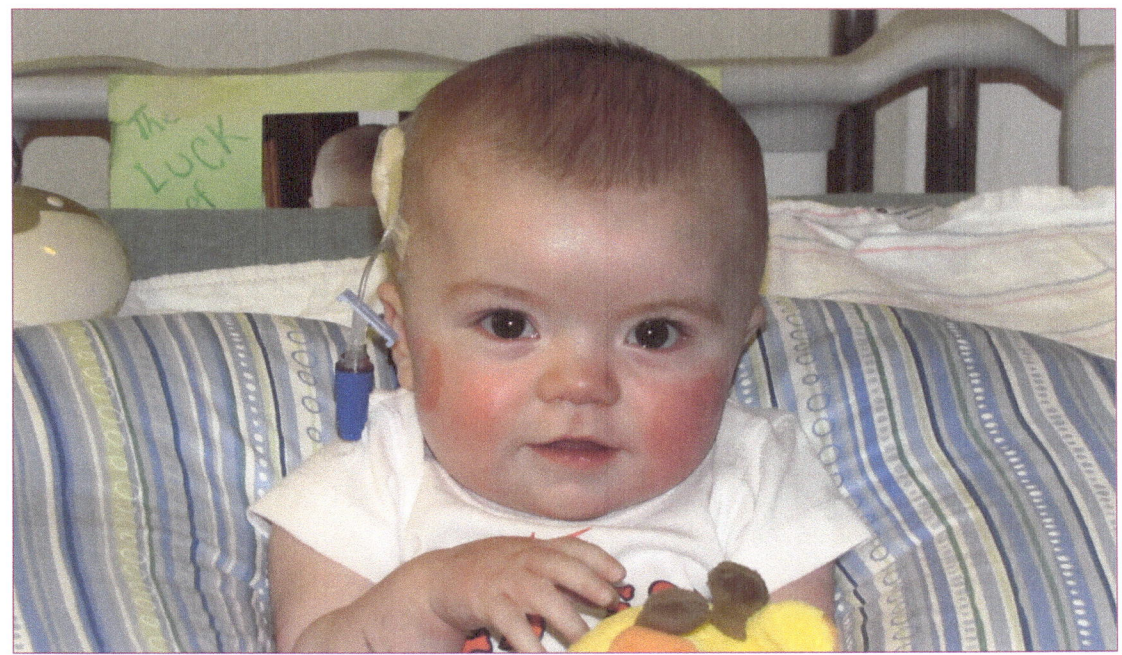

Lucas, on cardiology floor after Glenn operation

THIRD STAGE OPERATION FOR SINGLE VENTRICLE DEFECTS:
FONTAN PROCEDURE

Your child will need further imaging tests and a cardiac catheterization or MRI before the Fontan surgery and may have to spend the night in the hospital afterwards. The purpose of the catheterization is to measure the pressures and function of the heart and do interventions if needed.

Preparation for the Fontan surgery will include a one-day outpatient pre-operative assessment by our cardiology and cardiac anesthesia team. Your child's exact plan will be explained in detail to you.

The Fontan procedure can only work if blood flows passively at low pressure through the lungs since there is no ventricle to push it through. At birth, the blood pressure in a baby's lungs is high and decreases slowly over the first year of life. This is why the first and second stage operations need to be performed before the Fontan procedure.

The Fontan procedure guides the blood flow coming back from the lower body into the lungs without the help of a pumping chamber. The operation takes advantage of the fact that blood flows so easily through the lungs that it does not need the force of the right ventricle to push it through. The large vein bringing blood back from the lower body (called the inferior vena cava) is connected to the pulmonary artery, just as was done with the vein from the upper body (called the superior vena cava) during the bidirectional Glenn operation.

The Fontan procedure connects the inferior vena cava to the pulmonary artery by making a channel (also called a baffle) through the atria of the heart to direct its flow to the pulmonary artery. Sometimes a tube can be placed just behind the heart to make this connection (an extra-cardiac conduit). To

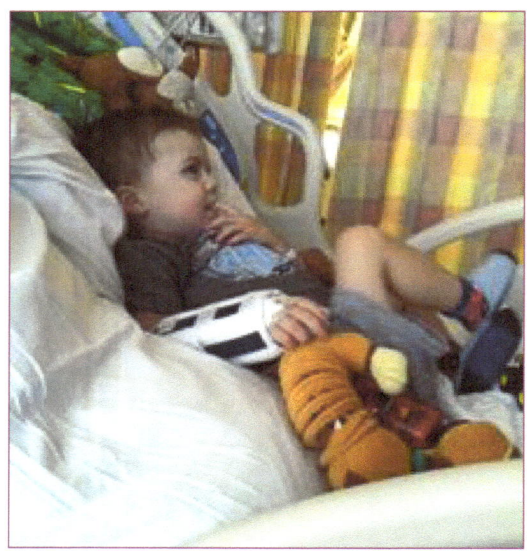

Lucas, on cardiology floor after Fontan operation

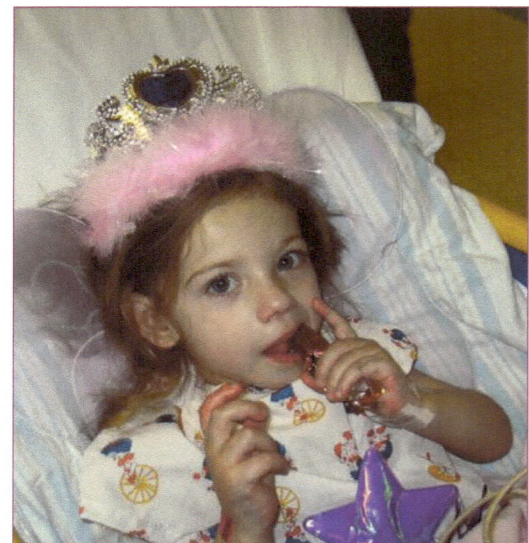

Grace, celebrates Halloween on the cardiology floor after Fontan operation

prevent sudden build-up of pressure in this pathway immediately after surgery as the body adjusts to the new blood flow patterns, a small "pop-off" hole (also called a fenestration) is made. This fenestration may close on its own, or may need to be closed with a device during a cardiac catheterization procedure many months or years later.

After the Fontan procedure, blue blood goes straight to the lungs through connections of the superior vena cava (done in the second stage surgery) and the inferior vena cava (done in the Fontan surgery) to the pulmonary arteries. Blood picks up oxygen in the lungs and returns as red blood to the single ventricle from which it is pumped to the body. The blood flow is now separated; red blood and blue blood no longer mix in the ventricle, so all the organs of the body (including the heart) receive better oxygen supply to function.

Average age at time of surgery: 18 months to 4 years; timing will depend on the unique needs of your child.

Expected hospital stay: one to three weeks. This is usually a more intense recovery than the bidirectional Glenn surgery. Children often spend two to four days in the CICU after surgery and then the rest of their stay on the cardiology floor. A common post-operative problem is pleural effusion: a buildup of fluid around the lungs. Pleural effusions may require drainage through chest tubes until the fluid production slows down.

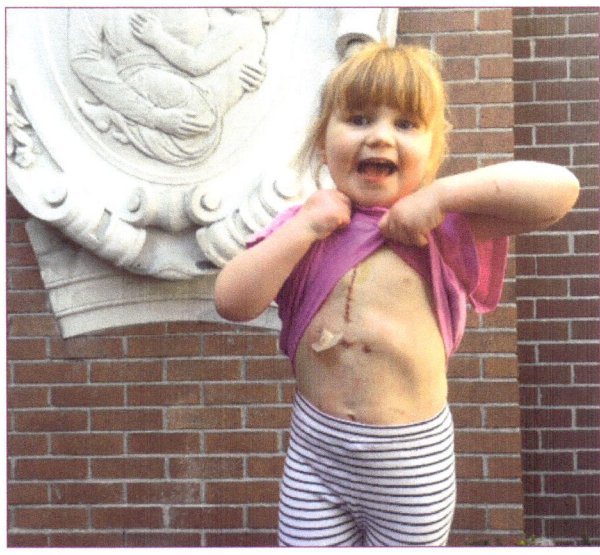

Mila, leaving the hospital after Fontan operation

Children also receive diuretic medicines (medicines to help remove extra fluid) due to fluid shifts. Another common post-operative problem is fast or slow heart rates that may call for medicines or pacing for a short time.

This is also a more challenging recovery because of the developmental stage of toddlers and preschoolers. Developmentally, your child may be more fearful and have limited skills to understand and express concerns. Physical discomfort, disruption in normal routine and sleep patterns, and required monitoring may increase discomfort. Many parents ask when they should start to talk to their child about the upcoming surgery. In general, it is best to wait a few days before

surgery. This can also be applied to siblings. Our Child Life Team (617-355-9410) is on hand to help you prepare your child for surgery.

Oxygen saturation levels: When fully recovered from the Fontan operation, most children have an improved oxygen saturation level above 85 percent. This will increase after the fenestration (small hole) is closed, which may happen naturally on its own, or after a catheterization procedure performed several months or years later.

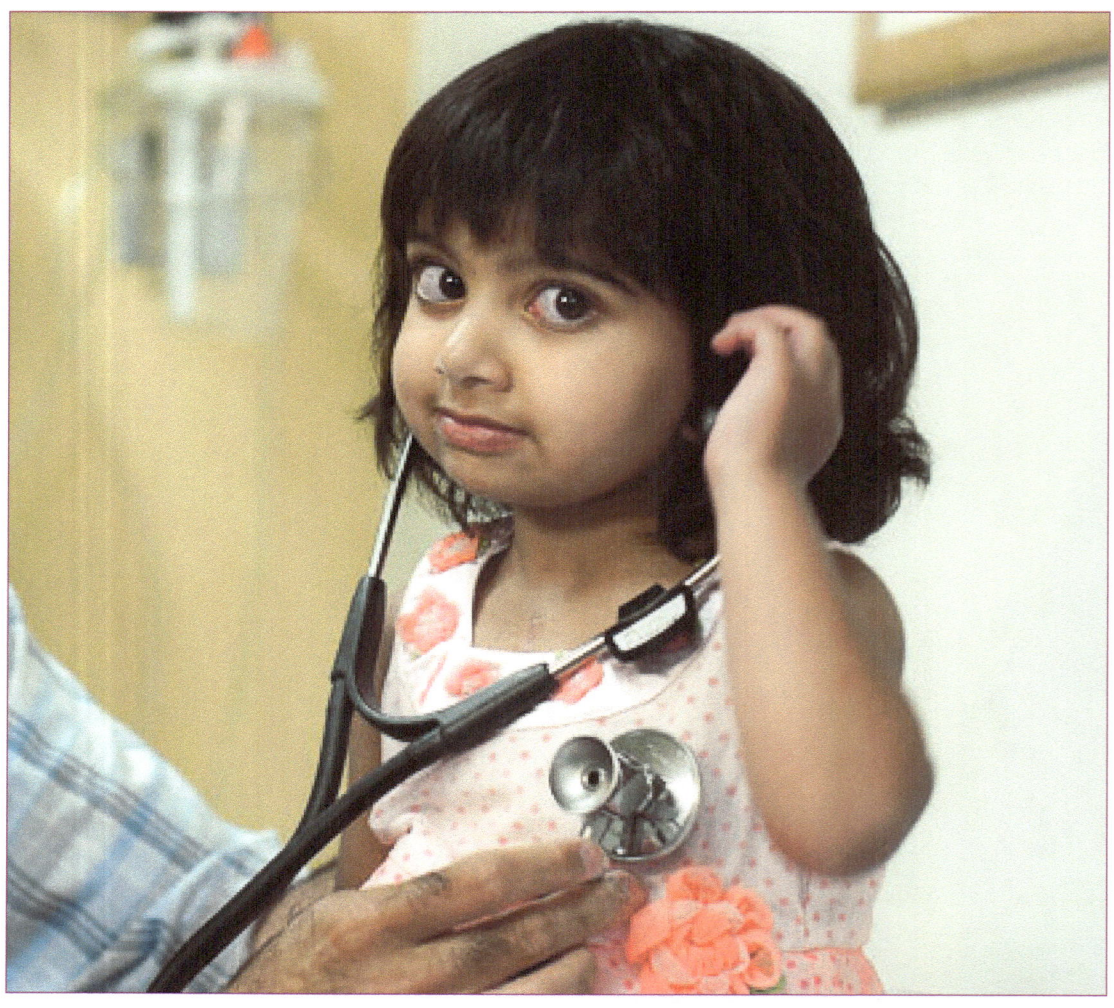

Catherine, at cardiology clinic visit after Fontan operation

PREPARING TO TAKE YOUR BABY HOME AFTER THE FIRST SURGERY

What goals will my baby need to meet before leaving the hospital?

Once your baby is transferred to the cardiology floor, there will be many recovery goals to meet before going home. The time on the cardiology ward may be longer than the time in the CICU and can sometimes be the most taxing on tired parents.

We have outlined your baby's expected goals below, and have made a "Roadmap to Home" (see page 33).

Goal 1: Stable heart and lung status. By the time your baby arrives on the cardiology floor, their heart and lung status will be more stable, but close monitoring with daily physical exams and changes in medicines are still needed. At first, your baby may be given oxygen through a nasal cannula, which gives oxygen right into the nostrils. In most cases, the amount of oxygen will be slowly decreased until your baby is safely breathing room air.

Before going home, your baby will have a final echocardiogram, chest x-ray, blood work, and an electrocardiogram to give an updated picture of heart and lung health.

Goal 2: Learn to eat and gain weight. (See Growth and Nutrition section for more information, on page 34).

Learning to eat
One of the biggest challenges your baby will face during recovery is learning how to eat so he or she can grow. At first, your baby will get breast milk or formula through a nasogastric tube (a small tube that runs from the nose to their stomach). We will start breast- or bottle-feeding when your baby shows signs of readiness (comfortable breathing, alert, stable heart and lung status). This part of the recovery can be surprisingly slow and sometimes a challenging process because most babies did not have a chance to develop feeding skills before surgery and they often tire easily; feeding is a lot of work for them! Be patient, and remember your baby will have many chances to learn to co-ordinate sucking, swallowing and breathing during feeding because they eat every few hours.

Feeding-related problems
Many babies have problems with vomiting (throwing up) and irritability because of feeding troubles. Many babies also have gastro esophageal reflux disease (GERD) and milk protein sensitivity. They may benefit from different medicines or changes to your diet if you are breastfeeding and/or using special baby formulas. Some babies may need care from other specialists who can help them overcome feeding issues. Our caring, expert team will work with you to find the right approach to help your baby eat and gain weight well.

Goal 3: Taking care of other health issues. Your baby may have other health issues—common in newborns—that need assessment or care during the recovery phase. They may have other congenital anomalies that need evaluation or treatment. There may be problems that occurred after surgery that

"If your child is progressing in the right way, going from CICU to cardiology floor will feel like you are all on your own. This is a good thing! The ICU feels very comforting, because there is a nurse at your baby's side at all times. When you are moved from ICU to 8 East, and the nurses and doctors only come check up on you every few hours, you may feel very alone at first. In our case, this was our first baby, so we truly did not have any experience in any aspect of taking care of her." Mila's parent

continue to need treatment. Many babies need to be slowly weaned off sedative and pain medicines provided during their time in the CICU in order to minimize symptoms of withdrawal.

Goal 4: Parent education. Before your baby goes home, we will offer you the guidance and education you need to feel comfortable taking care of your baby at home. Please review the "Roadmap to Home" for a checklist of items. It is never too soon to start learning about your baby's needs.

What is the Home Monitoring Program?

The time between the First and Second Stage surgeries is a very important period for your baby. The heart circulation is less stable than it will be after the second stage surgery and there is higher risk for infections, poor growth and other health issues during this time. Boston Children's Home Monitoring Program was started to support you during this challenging time. You will be given detailed guidelines and goals for your baby's growth and oxygen saturation levels, and will be supplied with a pulse oximeter (a painless sensor device that measures oxygen levels in the blood), baby digital scale and a notebook to record your baby's daily information.

We will give you instructions, tools and "red flags" to look out for so that you can call your treatment team if you spot a possible problem. Also, you will have weekly phone or email contact with a nurse practitioner who will review your baby's health with you. We will talk about the Home Monitoring Program with you in detail before your baby goes home. We will work closely with your local caregivers, your Boston Children's cardiology team and other specialists involved in your child's care.

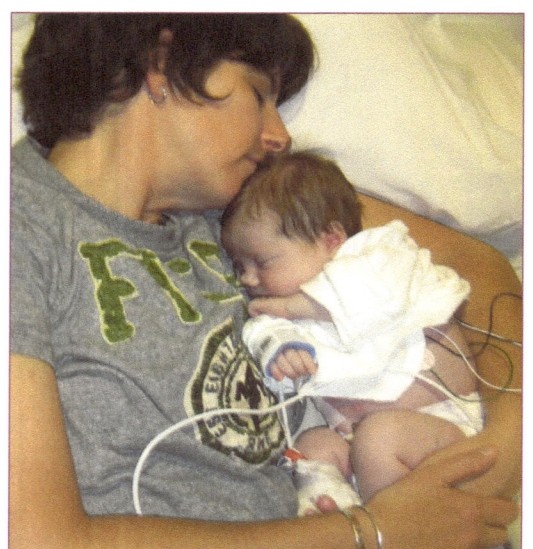

Kaya and mom, snuggling before discharge home

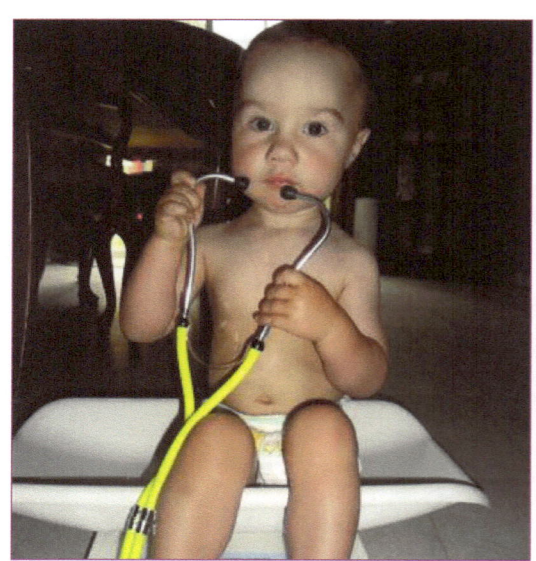

Parker, growing at home

Roadmap to home

General Care

☐	We can tell you about our child's heart condition and their surgery.
☐	We know what is expected of us during the post-op stay on 8 East.
☐	We have received the Newborn Teaching Packet and have reviewed it.
☐	We have completed: 　，PKU Screen 　，Hearing Screen 　，Car Seat Challenge 　，All Babies Cry 　，CPR
☐	We have received the post-op teaching sheet and know how to care for our child's incision at home.
☐	We know when to call the doctor and when to call for emergency help (911).
☐	We have stayed overnight with our child and cared for them for 24 hours. (*One parent is encouraged to stay at the bedside so you can participate in care and receive the teaching and education you need to care for your child at home.*)
☐	We know who the Social Worker, the Resource Specialist, and the Child Life Specialists are and we understand what they do.

Medications

☐	We can tell you what medications our child takes and why our child takes them.
☐	We can tell you the times and doses of our child's medications.
☐	We have practiced drawing up medications with the nurse.
☐	We have practiced giving medications to our child.
☐	We have our prescriptions and found a compounding pharmacy if needed.
☐	We have picked up our medications for home before discharge and reviewed them with the Nurse or Nurse Practitioner.

Feeding

☐	We know how to feed our child and have practiced giving them a bottle.
☐	We know who the Dietitian and/or Lactation Specialist is and how to call them.
☐	We know what calorie formula or breast milk our child is on.
☐	We know how to prepare breast milk/formula and have talked with the Dietitian about milk preparation.
☐	We have our formula and additives to increase the calories.
☐	We know how much our child should be eating in a day. If our child falls below the goal, we know to call the Home Monitoring Team.

Outpatient Support and Follow-Up

☐	We know who our Home Monitoring Team is and what they do. We know how to contact the team and when to call them.
☐	We have completed our home monitoring teaching and have demonstrated the ability to: 　，Use the scale and weigh our baby 　，Use the pulse oximeter 　，Fill out our Home Monitoring Log Book
☐	We know who our Visiting Nurse Agency is and how to contact them.
☐	We know who our home supply company is and how to get in touch with them. If we were given equipment from our home supply company, we know how to use it.
☐	We have met the Cardiac Neurodevelopment team.
☐	We made an appointment with our home Cardiologist to be seen within 2 weeks.
☐	We made an appointment with our home Pediatrician to be seen within 2 weeks.
☐	We know the plan for immunizations and for RSV prophylaxis (Synergist).
☐	We know how to contact Early Intervention Services.
☐	If needed, we have the contact information of other specialists our child needs to see and have made appointments to follow-up with them.

GROWTH AND NUTRITION

Can I breastfeed my baby?

If you planned to breastfeed your baby before you learned of your child's cardiac diagnosis, this plan does not need to change. If you were unsure about your feeding choice, talk to a lactation consultant about the many benefits your milk can give to your baby because of their added medical needs. Breast milk is an important part of your new baby's health care management. We encourage you to share this vital nutrition only you can give to your baby.

Even if your baby cannot eat right away, you can express your milk with a breast pump to save for later use. Breast milk can be fed through a feeding tube until a baby is strong enough to eat by mouth. Many babies with single ventricles need extra calories added to their feedings to help them grow and this is can be done by adding high calorie supplements to your breast milk for bottle or tube feedings.

The lactation consultants and nursing staff will be on hand to help you establish your milk supply with a breast pump and help you teach your baby how to breastfeed. Some babies can start to practice breastfeeding on a recently pumped breast for non-nutritive sucking to help develop breastfeeding skills. Often a combination of breastfeeding and breast milk by bottle with extra calories can meet the baby's needs. Some babies are eventually able to transition to breastfeeding with success.

What are the benefits of breast milk?

» contains immune properties to help fight infections

» lowers the risk of the bowel condition called Necrotizing Enterocolitis (NEC)

» is easily digested and better tolerated by the baby's stomach and intestines

» improves baby's development and neurological outcomes

Will my baby have issues with feeding and growing?

Good nutrition is linked to better surgical and developmental outcomes. Your baby will also need more calories and nutritional support because of their heart defect. Our goal is to give your baby enough nutrition to allow close to normal growth.

"I had successfully breastfed five healthy children. We learned that our sixth child, Peter, had HLHS in utero. One of my concerns was will he be able to be to breastfeed? I learned that feeding this baby will most likely be nothing like feeding my other children. Meaning, it was very common for these babies to have feeding issues and not to get my hopes up. As Peter's birth approached, I just assumed that breastfeeding would not happen. But, I was going to try anyway! Peter's first attempt at breastfeeding occurred when he was 2 weeks old. The first few attempts he was a bit sleepy and trying to figure it all out. We did not give up! He and I just stuck with it. In a few days, he had it all figured out and was doing great! His feeding tube was removed and he was not drinking from any bottles. I was excited to learn it was exactly like feeding my other babies! He was discharged from the hospital with the nutrition plan of exclusively breastfeeding. He has done wonderfully and has never run into any feeding or reflux issues. It is good to know that there is hope. Hope does not mean that you are not accepting that things may not go as you'd like them to go. Hope just gives you strength to get through your difficult situation." Peter's parent (see picture on page 35).

We will watch your baby's growth and nutrition status carefully during the hospital stay and after going home. We have a dedicated registered dietician on our team. She will help decide how many calories your baby needs to eat per day and teach you how to increase the caloric density of your breast milk or make formula if needed. She will be on hand during the first hospital stay and will be in contact with you by phone or email between the first and second stage surgeries to make sure feeding and growth stays on track.

To overcome feeding issues, some babies may need care from other specialists such as gastroenterologists, pulmonologists, ear nose and throat specialists, feeding specialists and occupational therapists. Together, we will work to find a way to help your baby thrive.

What are the potential feeding and growing issues?

1) Gastro esophageal reflux disease (GERD)

At either end of your esophagus (feeding tube from your throat to your stomach) is a small sphincter (muscle ring) that is held together by ligaments from the diaphragm. The ligaments holding the baby's sphincter are undeveloped, the esophagus is shorter, and infants lie down much of the time. This, combined with cardiac problems, can increase the chances of mild to severe reflux, which can create a painful burning feeling due to the contents of the stomach backing up into the esophagus. GERD symptoms can include crying and irritability, poor eating and vomiting (throwing up). When babies have pain or cry, but do not spit up or vomit, reflux can still be there. Babies with GERD may benefit from different medicines or other changes that we will discuss with you.

2) Milk protein allergy

GERD may also be a symptom of **milk protein allergy** which is when the baby has difficulty digesting large protein molecules (such as milk, soy and egg) because their immune system is immature and mistakenly reacts to the proteins as if they are germs, essentially causing an allergic reaction. This is not the same as lactose intolerance (not making the enzyme needed to digest the sugar found in milk). Symptoms of milk protein allergy include: irritability (which can look like colic); reflux; slow weight gain; gas; stomach pain; loose, runny, stool that is green or contains mucus or blood; constipation (hard poop); rash (dry skin, eczema, or cradle cap). These babies often tolerate breast milk better than formula because it is easier to digest. Typically, a milk allergy goes away by the time a child is 1 or 2 years old. If a milk protein allergy is suspected, we will talk about treatment with you. Breastfeeding moms are encouraged to follow a milk/soy/egg elimination diet and formula-fed babies will be changed to a special formula that is easier to digest.

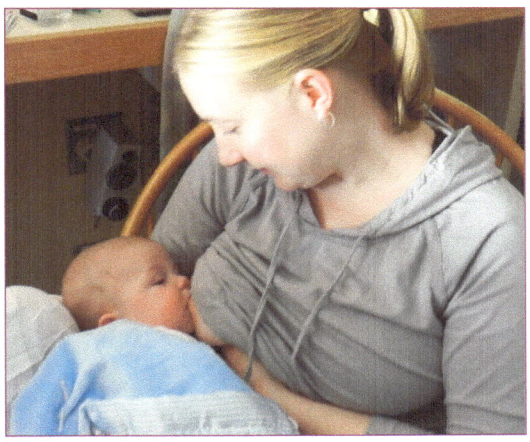

Kerri, nursing baby Peter who is recovering from Glenn operation for HLHS

3) Other issues

Your baby may also need to switch to a modified fat breast milk or a special low fat formula for a short time if they get **chylous effusions** (milky-looking fluid building up or draining from around the lungs).

About 30% of single ventricle babies may not be able to breast- or bottle-feed all of the calories needed to grow. This could be due to **oral aversion** (not liking anything in or around the mouth), **vocal cord dysfunction** (injury to a vocal cord nerve causing soft cry or swallowing difficulties), or not having enough strength to eat all required calories by mouth. To give nutrition while your baby is learning to eat by mouth, we may suggest other ways of feeding such as placement of a gastrostomy tube (G-tube, see picture on page 37), which is a feeding tube placed through the skin over the belly that gives nutrition straight to the stomach. Your baby may benefit from using this while learning to breast- or bottle-feed. We will talk about the option more in detail with you if we think it would be helpful for your baby.

Other parent experiences

We recently surveyed a group of parents with babies who were born with single ventricle heart defects. The topic they wished they had more preparation for was "feeding and growing." Here are some personal stories from these parents who have had firsthand growth and nutrition issues. The aim is not to frighten you, but to share information from other parents about some of their feeding experiences. This does not mean your baby will necessarily have these problems.

Reflux

"I had a hard time with the fact that no matter how hard I tried sometimes my baby just wouldn't eat (due to reflux and allergies). and that it's hard to accept that your breast milk isn't enough to make your baby grow." Kane's parent

"Reflux!! Holy cow I was not prepared for reflux. I had no idea it was such a huge problem. Reflux is what nearly broke us. Once we made changes, things got much better." Addie's parent

"Reflux has been the biggest hurdle by far. There is nothing sadder than your little baby throwing up. I'm pretty sure I cried more than she did about it. Prilosec and Zantac have been our best friends, as well as a reclining chair to sleep in at night during the first few months. Elevating her crib is now key, and we hold her upright for at least 30 minutes after she eats during the day." Genevieve's parent

Oral aversion

"Since Brooklyn was NPO (nothing by mouth) for essentially five months, the road to oral eating was inevitably going to be difficult, although I honestly had NO idea how difficult it would really be. From the first day, we kept her sucking on the pacifier and she had a really strong suck. Hence, I didn't think it was going to be difficult. She had her Glenn procedure at 5 months old. She went into the Glenn sucking away on the paci-

"All babies, including those with serious heart disease, have an important plumbing system in their body called their gastrointestinal (GI) tract that has to be working well if they are going to be happy and totally healthy. Tuning this plumbing system up by softening stools, changing diets and treating acid reflux —if a baby is suffering from any or all of these issues—may be critical to finally helping them feel well enough to eat comfortably and grow. You may wonder how stool softeners (such as MiraLAX ®) can help with a baby's reflux. When a baby has to work—or "push to poop"—they can develop reflux. Often this occurs during feeding, which may make the baby cry during feeding or want to stop eating. By making stools soft, the baby does not have to push hard to poop so the reflux episodes are less. Also, remember, that babies can have silent reflux. Reflux does not only mean spitting up." Dr. Jenifer Lightdale, MD, MPH (Gastroenterologist)

fier, and she came out of the Glenn wanting NOTHING to do with it. Our soothing mechanism and our only path to oral eating was gone. Her gag reflex was heightened. For the next 8 months, it was a fight to get to her mouth and when we did it was a gag and vomit session. We started with Occupational Therapy and Early Intervention right after we got home from the Norwood procedure and have had it 2 times a week since. At 13 months old, we had a breakthrough for about 2 weeks. She would take yogurt by the spoonful and swallow with no trouble. Two weeks later, she went back to the mouth being a "no entry zone." She has been drinking water and apple juice from a sippy cup since about 10 months old so liquid was never an issue. I couldn't make this up if I tried, but the week we started the "blenderized" diet she started put things in her mouth WILLINGLY! A month and a half after starting the new food, she started eating Gerber Puffs, Goldfish, Pirates Booty, Veggie Sticks, Cheerios and she is VERY interested in pizza and buttered bagels. We still have a LONG way to go until she understands the "chew, move it around your mouth and swallow" sequence. We still have some gagging issues but she wants to eat, and that is a HUGE difference."
Brooklyn's parent

Milk, soy, protein allergy

"Haven had developed a food allergy to milk and soy at around 4 months old. The most devastating thing about this was having an entire freezer full of pumped breast milk (and all the blood sweat and tears that went into it, literally) that I couldn't use. It was a super-upsetting experience to not be able to use it, let alone having to start pumping all over again on a milk-and-soy free diet. Awful! I did donate the eight gallons of breast milk to the Ohio Milk Bank—but it was very difficult to separate myself from the breast milk because pumping at the hospital during the first months of Haven's life literally felt like the ONLY thing I could do to help her. It's also super hard to eat a milk, soy and egg free diet at the hospital and when you are already stressed, exhausted and trying to pump, adding limitation to your diet is very stressful. A lot of the shopping and cooking became so complicated that I had to have a lot of help from family to stay healthy enough/well fed to keep up my energy level to keep pumping. It sincerely took a village to keep me up and running on this diet, along with managing hospital life, stress and Haven's condition. Thankfully, she's incredibly healthy today." Haven's parent

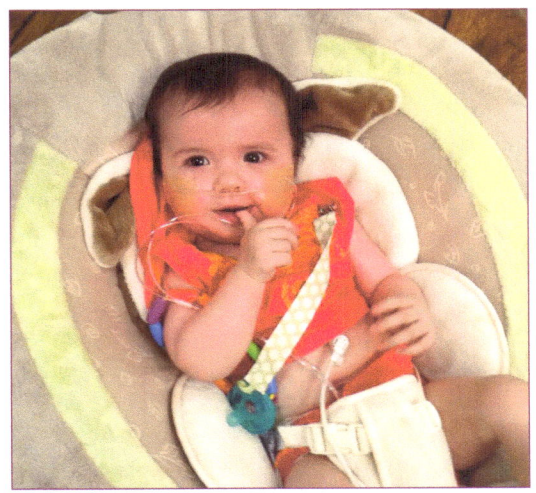

Baby Mary with G-tube on abdomen, which helped her grow close to the top of the growth charts!

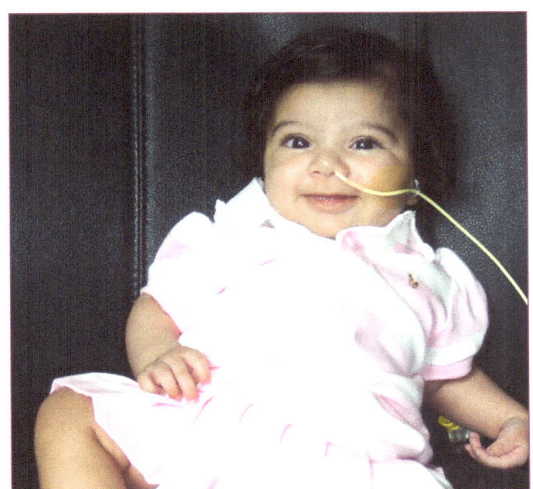

Baby Catherine, looking chubby thanks to the NG feeding tube

G-tube

"The G-tube was hands down the best decision we made for Genevieve. Being born slightly preterm and having had a lengthy intubation post op her Norwood led to a very slow start at eating. About 4 weeks post op when she was still getting fed through a NJ tube with no interest at all in eating, my husband and I were easily sold on the option of have a G-tube placed. It was an easy procedure and had us out of the hospital significantly earlier than if we had chosen not to have it placed... I'm pretty sure we would STILL be there if it hadn't been placed and she's now 5 months. The great thing about it is she can still work on oral feeds every day without the pressure of feeling she needs to finish in order to gain. Plus, I can put all of her meds through it which has helped avoid adding to her already present oral aversion." Genevieve's parent

Chylous effusions

"Shortly after our son's first surgery, the nurses noticed some fatty material in his Blake drains. These are tubes that come out of your child's chest and dispense into plastic pouches. The pouches, which hold extra fluid that is drawn from the chest cavity and off of the lungs, typically contain what looks the color of blood. In our son's case the fluid began to look milky and have large chunks of fat in it. These are called chylous effusions. It means that during surgery our son's lymphatic system was disturbed. The lymphatic system breaks down fats so that excess fluids can be drained or eventually passed through urine. However, if the lymphatic system is disrupted these fats cannot break down. Instead they will sit in the chest cavity. The largest impact of this information for me as a breast-pumping mom was that they removed my breast milk from his feeding tube and started him on a special formula. I urge mother's to remember that no matter what, nothing and no one can replace your role. If you are having emotional difficulty with a significant change like this, you can always ask to speak to an NP or request support. After he was switched to formula, we had to leave the drains in until they were clear. The surgeon chooses how long

that is. If you have questions about why he made his decision, you can always speak to the surgeon and ask him. The Blake drains are uncomfortable, but if your child seems to be in pain, you can speak to the nurses about pain management while they are in place. Your child will be on formula for 6 to 8 weeks. If you notice signs of a dairy or soy allergy, notify your NP or cardiologist. There are soy-free, dairy-free specialty formulas available such as Tolerex." Lucas' parent

Please note that we can now give babies modified fat breast milk in some cases.

Vocal cord paralysis

"After the Norwood procedure, we thought the worst was behind us. We were wrong. Dealing with our baby boy's feeding issues was beyond frustrating and heartbreaking. After many tests and tearful conversations with the doctors, we discovered he had a paralyzed vocal chord and was aspirating on all liquids. We had no choice but to send him into another surgery. He underwent the procedure for his PEG (feeding) tube about five weeks after his heart surgery. At the time, the idea of my child being fed through his stomach was scary and I thought it made him abnormal. Today, he is 7 months old and thriving. I have his PEG to thank for a lot of his progress!" Finn's parent

Poor weight gain and using breast hind milk (Hind milk is the high-fat, creamier milk towards the end of pumping or breastfeeding that the baby gets after the foremilk.)

"Our son was very uncomfortable while being fed fortified breast milk and oil, but he couldn't grow on straight breast milk. I worked with the lactation and nutrition teams at Boston Children's to spin the fat off of my breast milk and add it to my hindmilk to make 34 calories of naturally fortified breast milk. He is now feeling much better and gaining weight with this new technique. You may want to ask your team about this if your baby is uncomfortable on fortified formula or breast milk." Kalev's parent

Tips for feeding and what to talk to your team about

1. Ask for support if you want to breast-feed your baby. Ask to meet with one of our lactation consultants for help establishing a plan and schedule to keep yourself pumping milk regularly. This will keep up your milk supply and get your breastfeeding off to a good start. The consultants can be paged by your team to help you.

2. Bring your small amounts of early milk (called colostrum) to your baby's nurse. This can be used for mouth care and give early immune properties to your baby.

3. Bring a small cooler with an ice pack to help you store your milk.

4. Talk to your baby's team about how to practice breastfeeding as soon as your baby is able to feed by mouth.

5. Hold your baby skin-to-skin if you are able. This helps stimulate milk production, promotes bonding with your baby, and supports baby's development.

6. Use a breastfeeding pillow and ask about best positioning during breast and bottle feeds to keep you and your baby comfortable.

7. To support babies that are getting tube feedings:
   - Give your baby a pacifier during all tube feeds to help develop sucking skills.
   - Hold your baby during the feed to promote development, bonding and help with reflux symptoms.

8. Provide chin support to help support your baby during bottle feeding.

9. Learn your baby's feeding cues. If your baby appears to be hungry before the scheduled feeding, ask your nurse if you can feed your baby early. If your baby is very sleepy when the feed is ready, ask your nurse about delaying the feed for 30 minutes or so until your baby is showing "readiness to feed."

10. If your baby is not interested in feedings, not able to suck, or falls asleep after five or 10 minutes, it is best to stop the feeding and let them rest. Most of the time, trying to feed a baby for longer than 30 minutes can use up precious calories when your baby is trying to grow. There are at least eight feeds per day for your baby to learn to eat. Forcing your baby to eat could lead to other problems.

11. Remember to stop and burp your baby during the feeding.

12. Consider using low-flow nipples when you start bottle feeding.

13. Some positions are better after feeding to help avoid reflux. In general, after feedings babies should be held upright, placed in a bouncy seat, or in a crib with the head of the bed raised. Car seats can often make reflux symptoms worse.

For questions, please call the Boston Children's Hospital Lactation Support Program at 617-355-0005.

NEURODEVELOPMENTAL CONCERNS

Will my baby have problems with development and learning?

Recent research has suggested that children who have undergone heart surgery may have trouble developing their cognitive (thinking and information processing), motor and language skills.

Babies with single ventricles may have delays in reaching milestones like rolling over, crawling and walking. They may also have problems with feeding and sleeping routines. When older or beginning school, children may have issues with paying attention, acting impulsively or developing social skills. School-aged children often have academic struggles and may need extra support in the classroom. These issues can be minor problems that go away with time but may also be larger problems that need a lot of attention and support.

Finding out early and getting the right treatment are very important for these children. We strongly suggest that every child who has heart surgery be enrolled in an Early Intervention program that will provide therapeutic and support services designed to meet your child's individual needs. In addition, children with congenital heart defects are routinely evaluated by the Boston Children's Hospital Cardiac Neurodevelopmental Program.

See page 54 for tips on how to promote infant development in the hospital.

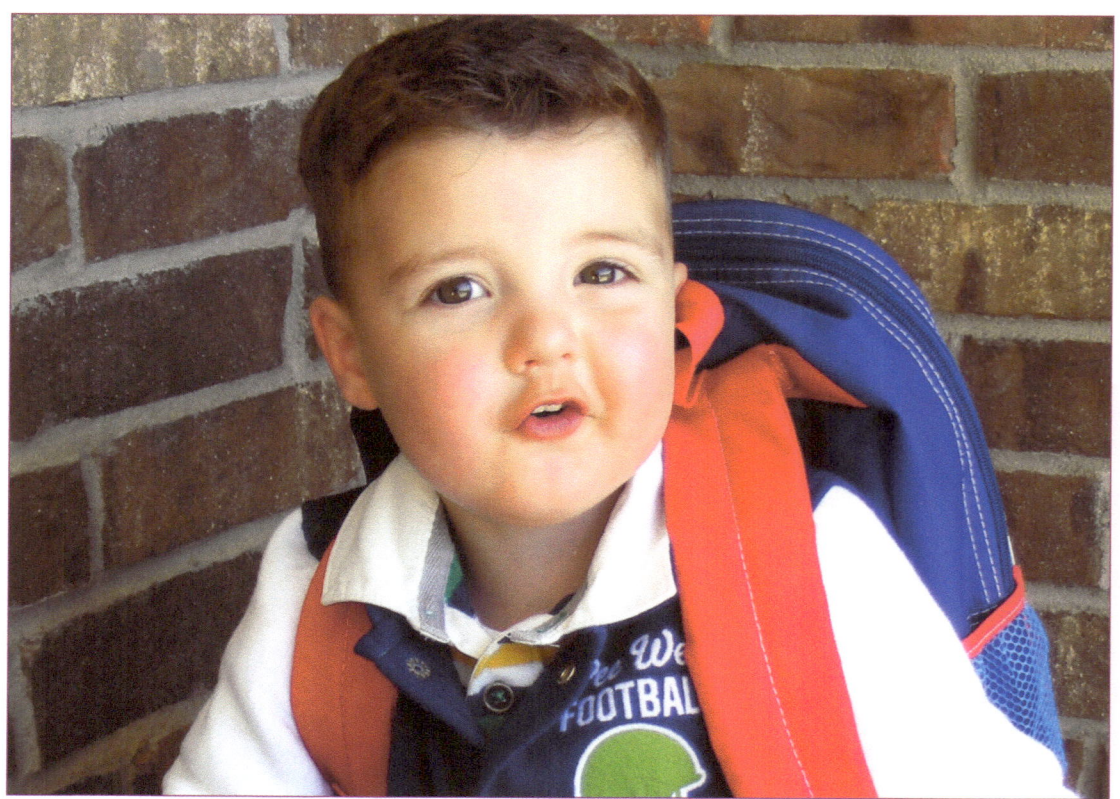

Sam, ready for school after Fontan operation

What is the Cardiac Neurodevelopmental Program?

This program—one of the first of its kind in the nation—emphasizes prevention through early detection and treatment of developmental delays. Team members work closely with parents, pediatricians and school personnel, and if needed, refer to treatment services tailored for each child.

Follow-up appointments with Boston Children Hospital's Cardiac Neurodevelopmental Program (CNP) are recommended at 6 months, 18 months and 36 months of age or sooner if needed. For appointments or questions for CNP, please call 617-355-3401.

"Being the parent of a child with HLHS has been the hardest and most rewarding thing I have ever done. Our daughter, Grace, is now 9 years old and doing so well —with so many thanks to Boston Children's Hospital. They have not only been there for our family through her heart journey; they are there for all of her (and our) needs! We are so fortunate for Grace to be doing so well medically. We now are in the part of our journey of a school-aged child with a serious cardiac condition. We also are all learning together how HLHS may affect her in terms of learning. Grace struggles in school academically, and nothing seems as easy for her as it does for her peers, but she always tries her hardest, and that is all we ask of her. She came into this world with sheer determination and faces every day with a smile. She continues to remind us to cherish every day. We are so blessed by our "Amazing Grace." Grace's parent

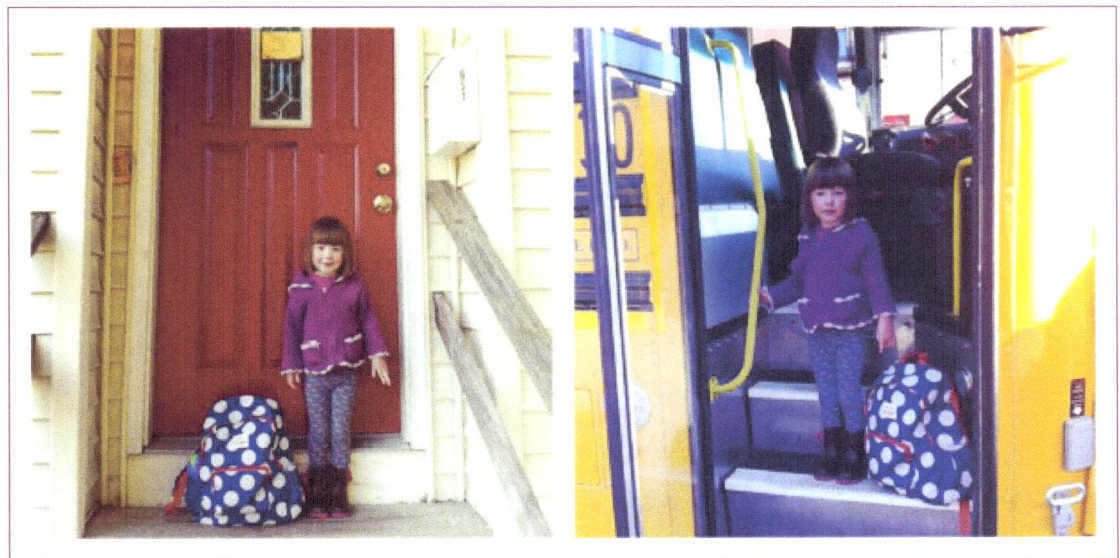

Haven, first day of preschool after Fontan operation

LONG-TERM OUTLOOK

What is the long-term outlook for my child?

It is not possible to predict the exact road, prognosis or life expectancy for your child. Your baby will never be cured of their heart defect and may need more surgeries or interventions in the future. They will live with a single ventricle circulation. All babies with single ventricle are unique, and some have more risk factors for later problems than others. Your cardiologist will talk about your baby's specific issues. Many children do well during the school-age years and may develop new health issues in the teen years.

Your child will always need to be cared for by a pediatric or adult cardiologist with specific expertise in congenital heart problems to watch for and treat any problems that come up. Such problems may include heart rhythms that are not normal, changes in liver function, blood clots, declining heart function (caused by weak heart muscle) and—as a result of all of this—challenges with day-to-day activities. At some point, your child may need to see other specialists who can help care for these problems, and it is possible a heart transplant will one day be needed.

"Having a baby born with a CHD is unimaginable. Whether we find out during pregnancy or after delivery, the shock of knowing our child isn't healthy is a feeling that is indescribable and at times unbearable. Zoe was diagnosed with HLHS at 18 weeks in utero.Thank heavens my husband and I found out before giving birth as we had several months to prepare. With eternal gratitude to the incredible nurses and doctors at Boston Children's Hospital, today our daughter is a walking miracle. Zoe just turned 11 years old, and she does gymnastics twice a week, runs, jumps, sings, dances and chases after her two little sisters. Our sweet girl is in school full time and for the most part knows her own limitations, understands that she needs extra water breaks and can't overdo it during the summer months. Zoe wears a bikini and loves to embrace the fact that she is a warrior with a zipper, proving she's been a survivor since the day she was born. Thanks to all of you, we have our daughter that continues to amaze us and bless us with her presence each and every day." Zoe's parent

---

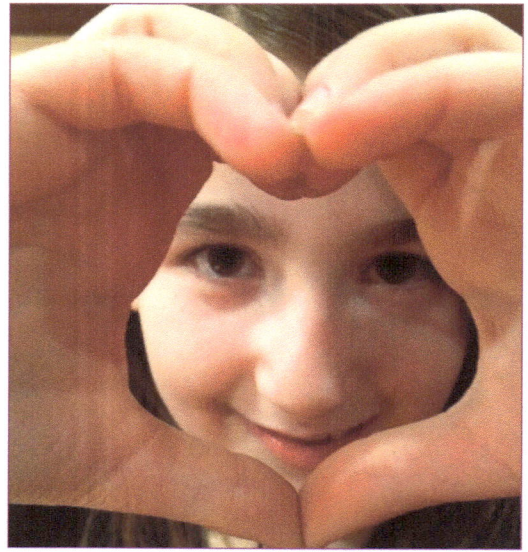

Zoe, now an energetic and happy teenager

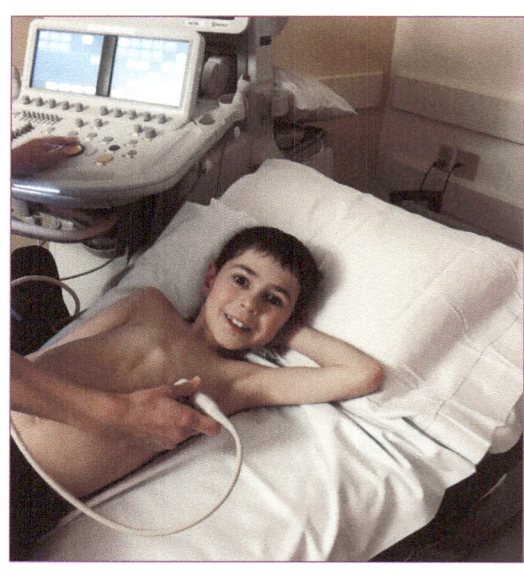

Joseph, in cardiology clinic for a routine echocardiogram

Successful operations performed on these babies have only been possible in the past 30 years, and there were only a small number of patients treated with these new procedures in the early years. There are few adults living with single ventricle heart defects who had surgery as infants, so we are just starting to learn more about how patients will do as they reach adulthood.

Many parents of daughters ask if they will be able to become pregnant. Some women with single ventricles have had successful pregnancies, but before pregnancy, we suggest a full cardiac evaluation by an expert adult cardiologist specializing in congenital heart defects, as well as a consultation with a high-risk obstetrician experienced in caring for women with complex congenital heart defects.

The Boston Adult Congenital Heart (BACH) Service at Boston Children's provides ongoing inpatient and outpatient care and advanced therapeutic options for patients with all forms of congenital heart disease as they progress into the teen years and adulthood.

The Adult Congenital Heart Association is a national, not-for-profit organization dedicated to improving and extending the life of adults with congenital heart defects, who now number more than one million. The organization serves and supports these adults, their families and the medical community. Learn more at achaheart.org.

"These heart kids are limited, and they innately have interests that align with their abilities. It's kind of like God creates them with the innate interests that are just perfect for them. Having Ethan has made our life better, richer; it changed us forever. We learned that there are things in life that are completely worthy of giving your all and then some to. My life without Ethan would be incomplete. Ethan inspires me each day, and I will never stop loving him, advocating for him and learning from him and his life. Even though the road is long and hard, these kids are such a blessing. If people will open their hearts to this gift, their hearts and lives will be fuller than they ever thought possible." Ethan's parent

---

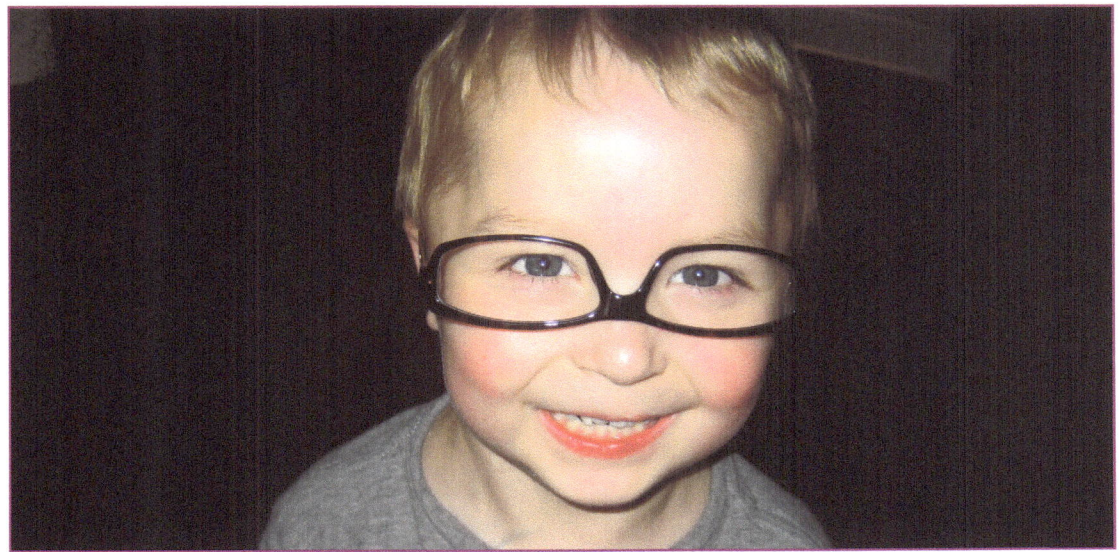

Ethan, smiling with his eyes and heart

Can my child take part in sports and exercise?

Most of our patients with Fontan circulation can dance, swim, ride horses, ride bicycles and play normally with their sisters and brothers. We encourage appropriate daily physical activity and a healthy, well-balanced diet to keep your child's heart as strong and healthy as possible. Exercise concerns or restrictions will be discussed in more detail as your child gets older.

Most children who have undergone Fontan surgery do not have normal exercise capacity and may have lower endurance levels. They can do most normal daily activities, but they may tire with more prolonged physical exercise like running, biking, skating, hiking and other strenuous activities. Your child will learn to set their own pace if an activity is too tiring and should be allowed to rest, eat snacks and drink water as needed.

"Having a daughter with "half of a heart" is scary and heartbreaking. The fear of the unknown is sometimes debilitating, but our young lady is full of love, light and hope. From one parent to another, stay strong, find hope and know that modern medical miracles happen every day."
Zoe's parent

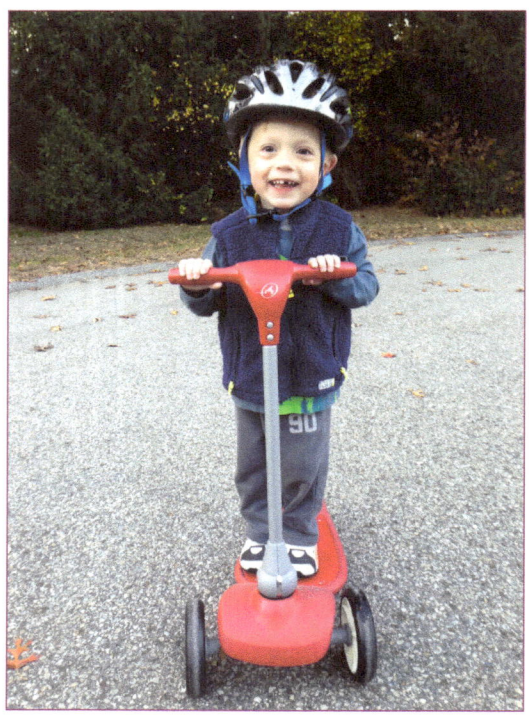

Kane, energetic and chasing his brother before Fontan operation for HLHS

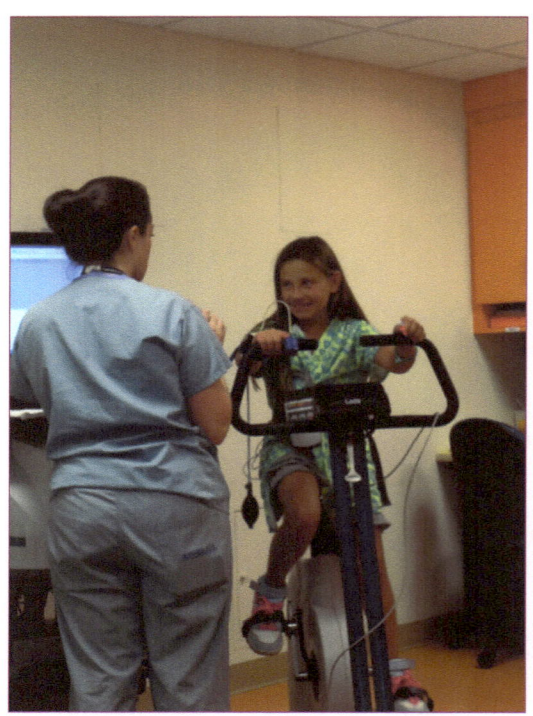

Grace, on exercise bike at clinic appointment

Will my child need a heart transplant?

For a small number of babies born with single ventricles, heart transplant is a better option than staged palliation. If needed, a multidisciplinary team will be involved in your child's care early on to help understand whether heart transplant would be feasible. However, most babies with single ventricle heart defects do not need heart transplants when they are babies or very young children. If your child experiences some of the complications of single ventricle anatomy, heart transplant may be a good option for them.

As your child gets older, the possible need for heart transplant increases. Although frightening at first, it is important to know that many children can do very well following heart transplant and can have normal activity, participate in sports, and thrive and grow. Boston Children's has an experienced heart transplant team that will meet with you to give you more information about this therapy. There are also other pediatric transplant programs throughout the country.

"We'll never say it will always be easy, but we will say it will all be worth it." Parker's parents

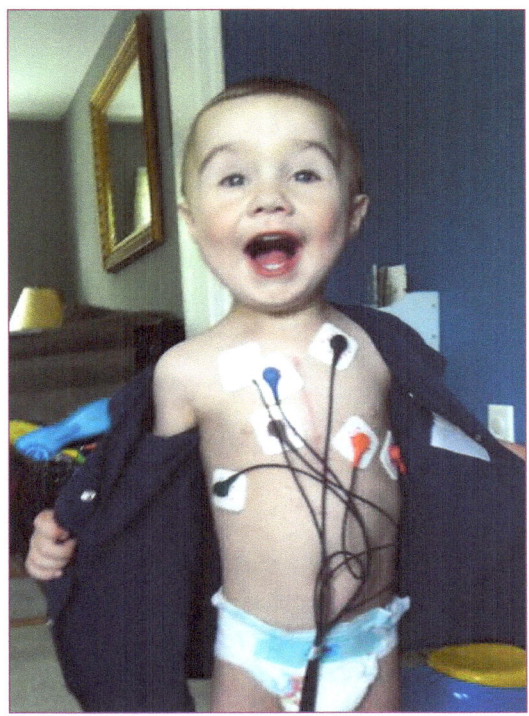

Parker, with Holter monitor

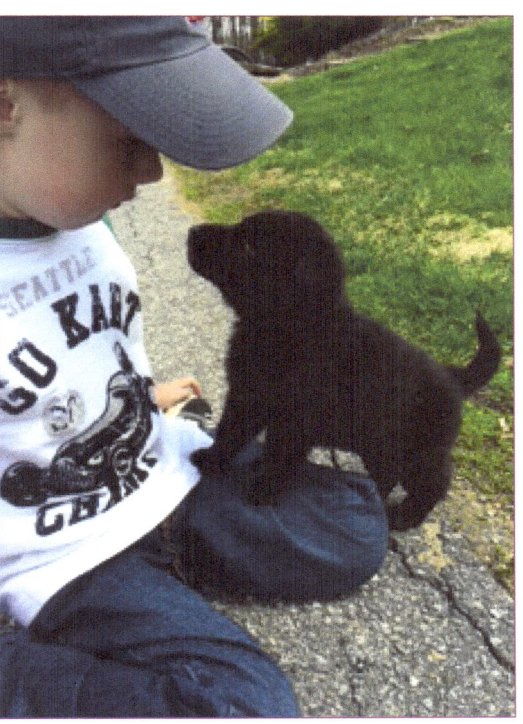

Parker, after Fontan playing with new puppy

Are there any heart-healthy tips I should keep in mind as my child grows?

Heart-healthy living is important at all ages. Like all of us, your child and their heart will benefit from a healthy diet, appropriate weight and an active, healthy lifestyle.

Also, please:

» Schedule your child for an appointment with a pediatric dentist at about 6 months of age. Children with congenital heart defects (CHD) are at higher risk for cavities and other dental issues that can impact growth and nutrition, speech development, and might increase the risk of heart-related infection. Cavities are preventable and reversible if treated at once. Ask how to take care of your child's oral health and when your child should start brushing and flossing. One choice for pediatric dental care is the Boston Children's Dental Office, 617-355-6571.

» Ask if your child should take antibiotics before seeing the dentist to protect against infection.

» Ask how secondhand smoke can affect your baby's heart and lungs.

» Ask how to set up heart-healthy nutritional habits early in life, and help your child learn to make healthy choices early on.

» Ask what are the right exercises for your child to build body mass and get fit.

» Ask about the safety of oral contraceptives (birth control pills) for your daughter when she grows older. Some types of birth control pills are unsafe for patients with CHD.

» Ask how to keep your child involved with their health care and how to promote autonomy to help them gain independence from you one day!

» Plan on talking to your child about how smoking, drugs and alcohol can harm their heart.

» Talk to your child about their heart condition and the medicines they need to take; help them learn more about their heart and how to keep it healthy.

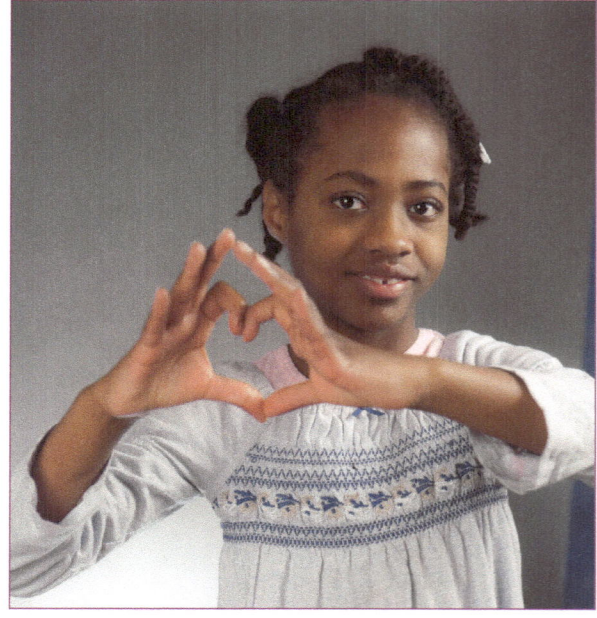

Grace Ann, celebrating her heart healthy living

What is the risk of having another child with HLHS?

In the case of children who have HLHS alone, recent studies have shown that their brothers and sisters have a greater chance (about 20 percent) of having a heart problem on the left side of the heart, which may range from a minor valve problem to HLHS. This chance slightly increases if one parent also has a left-sided heart defect. Because such heart problems can be very mild, parents may not know their child is affected unless they have an echocardiogram.

Screening recommendations
We suggest that brothers and sisters of children with single ventricle heart disease have a screening echocardiogram done when they are old enough to sit still for the test (so they will not need sedation).

If you become pregnant again, you should make an appointment for a fetal echocardiogram during your 18th week of pregnancy. You should also ask these questions during your first regular ultrasound appointment with your obstetrician:

» Do you see four chambers in the baby's heart?

» Are there two upper chambers with valves controlling blood flow into the heart?

» Are there two lower chambers with valves controlling blood flow out to the body?

» Do the valves and vessels leave the heart in a "crossing" fashion?

» Are the walls between the lower chambers of the heart intact?

» Is the baby's heart function normal?

In the case of a child who has single ventricle heart disease as well as additional abnormalities, there is an increased chance that he or she has a genetic syndrome. Whether future pregnancies would be at risk for the same syndrome depends upon the particular diagnosis. Your cardiologist can help you decide if your child should be evaluated by a clinical geneticist.

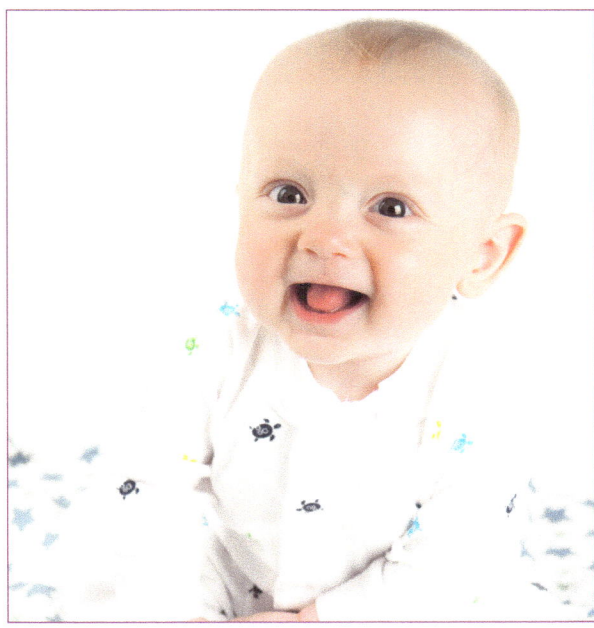

Baby Kane, before Glenn operation for HLHS

For this heart patient, what goes around, comes around

When Robin Scott was a little girl, traveling back and forth to the hospital to be treated for her single ventricle heart defect, her mother, Susan, had a simple wish: "What I really wanted was to see an older child who had a heart defect...I wanted to see teenagers, adults...I wanted to see people who had a normal life."

Funny how things work out. Today, Susan's daughter is 30 years old and working at Boston Children's Hospital—the same place she's been receiving treatment since she was born. Robin, who works in the Advanced Fetal Care Center (AFCC) is frequently asked to meet with fetal cardiac patients and their expectant parents, answering questions about her own experience and serving as a strong, healthy example of a congenital heart patient living a "normal" life.

Robin had volunteered at Boston Children's as a teenager and had "always wanted to work at the hospital." When a job opportunity came along in 2010, she took it. Strangely, Robin says that the job recruiters who helped place her at Boston Children's did not know that she had been treated there, and her personal history had nothing to do with their hiring decision.

Today Robin is often in contact with doctors and nurses who care for heart patients, and they regularly ask for Robin's help in answering questions from parents.

"When I speak to families, I always say each individual case is different," Robin explains, "but I do get a lot of the same questions: They ask, 'What were some of the challenges you faced growing up?' 'Did you play sports?' 'Did you date people?' They ask about my

scar. They ask about my parents' reactions."

What does Robin tell them? "I tell them about my own experience," she says. "I played sports—soccer and softball. I was a tomboy. The doctor never set any restrictions." She also expresses the importance of understanding your own condition and getting the support you need to stay healthy. "I was lucky to have two parents who were very present and very aware."

Being "present and aware" wasn't always easy. Robin's parents remember the difficulties they faced as she began her years of treatment. Susan remembers that right after Robin's birth, "the doctor said 'your daughter has a very serious heart defect, and she will certainly die if we don't perform surgery immediately.'" "It was the worst moment of my life, by far," Susan remembers. "I was always worrying. Why did it happen?" Her father, Tom, says that when Robin was born, "We didn't know anything. No one could tell us, they could never really assure us of anything."

Quickly, Tom and Susan learned as much as they could about Robin's specific heart condition (pulmonary atresia with intact ventricular septum), and they wondered what Robin's life—and their own—would be like. Susan credits the staff at Boston Children's for their support. "Dr. Freed was her cardiologist, and he let me ask anything, he was always available," she says. In addition, "the nurses in the clinic were wonderful."

Robin's parents say that they did not interact too often with other heart patient parents, stating that they were striving to treat Robin

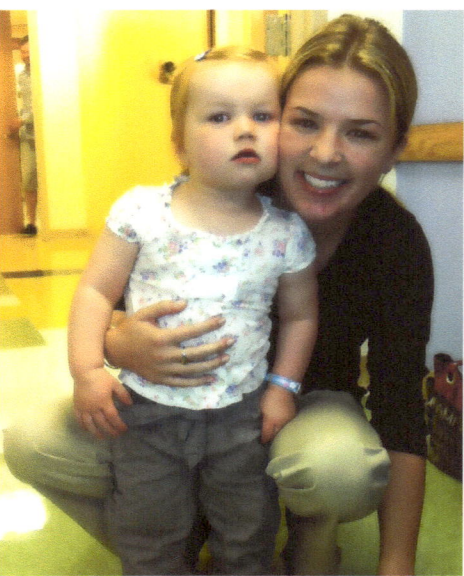

Mila (2) and Robin (30) became friends after learning they both have a form of hypoplastic right venricle

like a "normal" kid and not a kid defined by her condition. "My attitude from the start was that I didn't want her to feel that she was different, and I didn't want to feel different," Susan states.

Their approach seems to have worked. Robins asks, "Did I live a normal life? In terms of what normal is supposed to be, I feel that I did. Growing up, I knew that I was a little different, but I didn't think I had a disability."

Still, for Robin's parents, seeing an older heart patient, someone who had come through all the surgeries and treatments and was living a normal life, would have provided some comfort and hope over the years. "I would have loved to have had a Robin working in Cardiology—a 30-year-old woman who looks great," says Susan.

Today, heart patient parents at Boston Children's can meet that person in Robin Scott.

SUPPORT AND RESOURCES

How do I cope with the diagnosis?

Receiving the prenatal diagnosis that your unborn baby has a single ventricle heart defect is a major event for expectant parents. It can steal the joy from your pregnancy and cause you to question your dreams for your unborn child. Most importantly, it may force you to face a parent's worst nightmare: the prospect of losing your baby. You may recognize, for perhaps the first time, your inability to protect your child from all harm.

The journey after diagnosis is an extraordinarily hard time. You are grieving, yet you feel pressure to learn and prepare for your baby's arrival and any hard choices you must make. You may feel a rollercoaster of emotions until giving birth. Unlike your pregnant peers, your joy for this pregnancy may be tempered by worry and sadness. You may be reluctant to have baby showers or get a nursery ready until you know the baby is coming home. You and your partner may have different feelings, views or worries, and you may have relationship conflicts as a result. It may be helpful for you and your partner to talk with someone together about the stress of the diagnosis and how to emotionally prepare and cope with the road ahead.

Self-care after giving birth is vital. You have had a stressful pregnancy. You will likely be tired and uncomfortable from the delivery, and your own healing will mostly take place by your baby's bedside instead of in the

---

"All of the medical information as well as the breakdown of what to expect during the hospital stay is great, but one question that I desperately wanted answered was "What will our lives be like once this over?" When speaking with parents who are new to the CHD world, I tell each of them that LIFE WILL BE NORMAL. It may be a different type of NORMAL than you planned. No one plans on having a child with medical needs, but one day, everything will become second nature, and you will find yourself feeling normal. That big exhale that you have been waiting on since the day you found out your baby has a heart defect will come, and you will realize that you are all OK...changed, but better for it and most certainly normal." Addie's parent

---

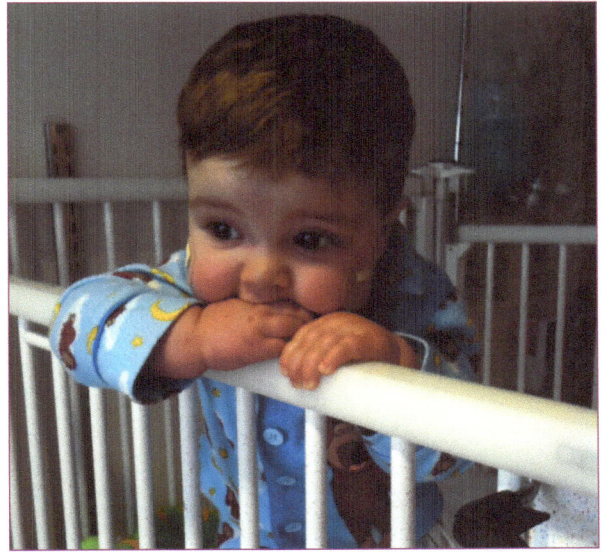

Sam, during an unexpected hospital stay

comfort of your own home. You may be nervous as you wait for the evolving plan of care for your baby. Post-partum mothers have fluctuations of mood. Be mindful of your mood, sleep and nutrition patterns. If you are not getting regular rest and proper nutrition, your ability to cope and think clearly will be diminished. If you need help, ask your obstetrician, social worker, or cardiology team. They are there to support you and your partner. You are not alone.

What do I tell my other children?

Our Child Life Specialists can help guide you in what to say and how to get your other children ready for your new baby and their heart condition. If you would like to speak with a Child Life Specialist before giving birth, please reach out to Maureen Abramson at 617-355-9410 or maureen.abramson2@cardio.chboston.org. You may also call the Office of Child Life Services at 617-355-6551.

"We wanted to get involved as much as we could and to arm ourselves with facts before our baby arrived. One of the ways we did that was to get enrolled in the annual "Little Hearts" picnic in Connecticut. We got connected to a few incredibly inspiring kids and very informative parents, with whom we are still in contact today. We were actually, surprisingly, the first family to ever go to the event while pregnant. We just wanted to know what we were in for before the surgeries began. It put things into perspective for us." Mila's parent

Ask for help

If you are feeling any of these symptons during your pregnancy or after your baby is born, please ask your obstetrician or any member of your baby's health care team for help:

- » Excessive tearfulness
- » Decreased appetite
- » Insomnia
- » Unrelenting worry
- » Nightmares
- » Aggitation or irritibility

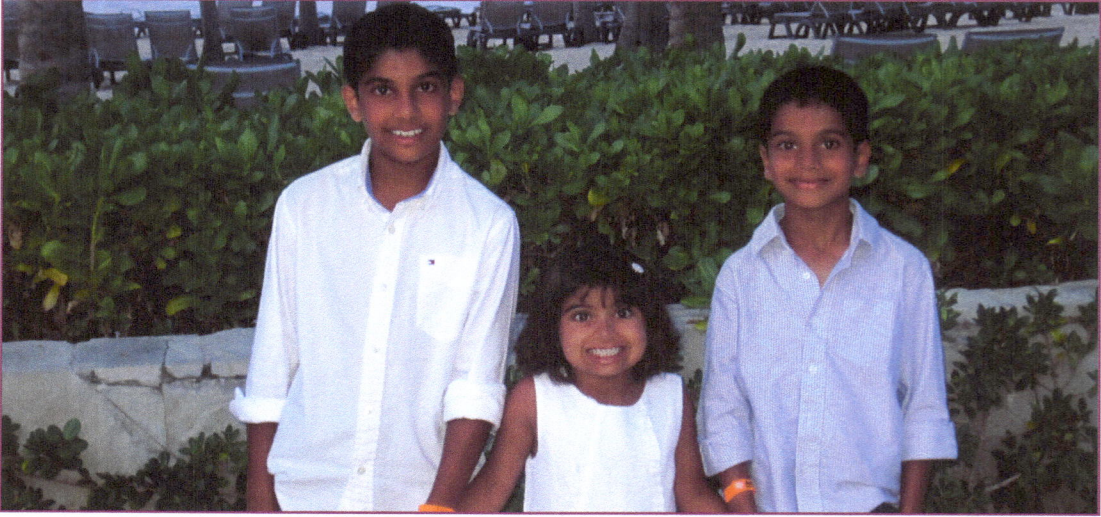

Catherine, enjoying her big brothers

Where can I find more information and support?

- » bostonchildrens.org/heart
- » facebook.com/heartcenter
- » mendedlittlehearts.org
- » heart.org
- » littlehearts.org
- » sisters-by-heart.org
- » linked-by-heart.org
- » childrensheartfoundation.org
- » jcchdqi.org

Another resource that may come in handy is Boston Children's MyWay (bostonchildrens.org/myway), a free mobile app with step-by-step directions to help you get around many hospital locations. It can also connect you with essential support services and give listings for kid-friendly activities and attractions in the Boston area.

In addition, many families have found that the book "Zip-Line" by David Humpherys is a lovely story written about a child that had open heart surgery and scar on their chest ("zip-line"). It may be helpful for siblings.

Sisters by Heart is a national parent support group involved in improving single ventricle outcomes

"Sisters by Heart was and continues to be a much needed support group for us. They are an amazing group of heart moms who are shoulders to lean on when no one else understands because they haven't been through it. These women have, and it makes them an invaluable resource to us along this incredible journey." Brooklyn's parent

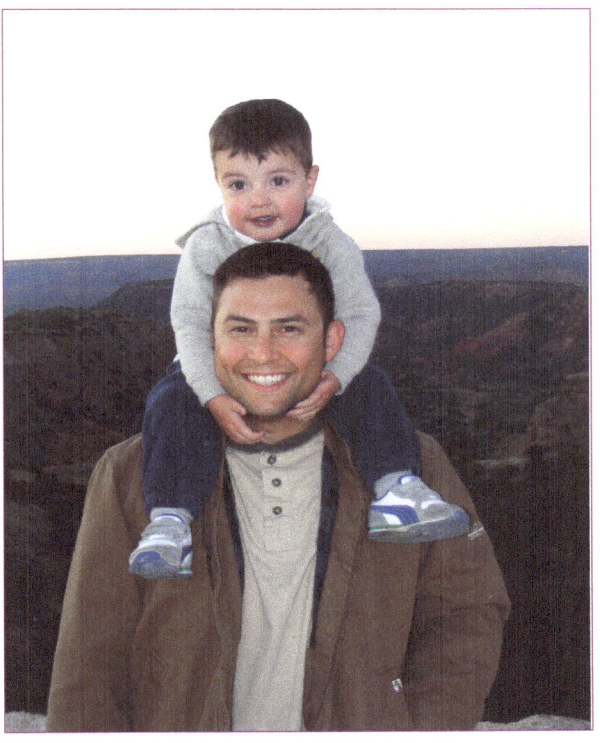

Sam and his dad exploring the world

WHAT TO BRING TO THE HOSPITAL FOR YOUR BABY'S FIRST OPERATION: A MOM'S RECOMMENDATIONS

Amber, the mother of a baby with hypoplastic left heart syndrome who was treated at Boston Children's, helped create this list:

» **12 x 12 blanket:** "We had a small square blanket for our baby, and the nurses used it all the time. It was a nice way to cover her since she couldn't wear clothes. I recommend bringing three in case they get dirty."

» **Baby-receiving blankets:** "They are prettier than the hospital blankets, softer and more personal. Once our baby was doing better, the nurses would cover her bed with the receiving blanket and then lay her on it. Then, they would cover her with the smaller 12x12 or swaddle her. While all of the other moms are at home placing their baby in the nursery they prepared for them, we heart moms need to make a nursery out of a hospital room. It was nice to see the things we had been given by loved ones wrapped around our baby."

» **Baby-wearing gear:** "A great way to calm fussy babies and promote bonding! The Moby Wrap is great, especially for small newborns that love to be held!"

» **Books, magazines**

» **Bouncy seat:** "To help with reflux issues or to help calm a fussy baby."

» **Bottles/nipples:** "The hospital provided bottles and nipples, but I wanted to use the kind I had at home. It never occurred to me to bring my own or buy some. If you want your baby to use a specific bottle-nipple combo, bring your own."

» **Breastfeeding pillow:** "This makes nursing or bottle-feeding your baby easier and more comfortable in the hospital. My Breast Friend Pillow provides more back support for mom."

» **Camera:** "I wish I had taken a picture of our baby with all of her nurses. They were all a blessing to us and will forever be part of her story."

» **Car seat:** "To leave the hospital in and to use for car seat test before discharge."

» **Chap stick:** "It can feel very dry in the hospital."

» **Clothes that are appropriate for the season in Boston:** It can get very cold in the winter and very warm in the summer, and sometimes the weather shifts dramatically from one day to the next. To be on the safe side, expect freezing cold snowy days in the winter and hot humid days in the summer.

» **Comfortable blanket**

» **Comfortable pillow:** "Sometimes the only way to escape from the stress is to try to sleep. A bad pillow will not help the situation. I know it sounds silly, but bringing a comfy pillow is something I wish I had thought of."

» **Create a Care Page or Caring Bridge Page** so you can more easily communicate with family and friends. They can also be used as a journal for yourself. Caring Bridge is available in English and Spanish.

» **Egg crate mattress:** "I think we spent three weeks sleeping in a chair. Bringing an egg crate mattress made a huge difference."

» **Going-home outfit:** "You'll want to take a ton of pictures!"

» **Measuring spoons:** "We stayed in Boston for a week after discharge and needed to measure her formula. We used a medicine cup, and it was not easy. Having a real tablespoon and teaspoon would have been wonderful."

» **Name and phone number for preferred pharmacy near your home**

» **Name and contact information for your pediatrician**

» **Name and contact information for your local cardiologist** (if needed).

» **Names and contact information of people you can ask for help**: "Here's some ideas of things to ask for help with: grocery shopping, caring for your other children, cooking meals, checking home for mail or security, cleaning and laundry, making or canceling appointments, making phone calls, driving or helping with transportation, caring for pets, staying with you at the hospital and staying at the bedside so that you can take a break."

» **Pictures of family:** "To post in room or on crib."

» **Planner or diary:** "A planner is always nice to document your child's overall health each day and track when dosages and medicines changed or stopped. You think you will remember, but you are so nervous. I wrote it all down and would always be looking through it. You feel like you have some control if you write things down, and I felt like I was somehow helping. Also, if you keep a diary, it can be a release to express emotions, and it can help later on when you look back at what you have been through."

» **Slip-on shoes:** "You lie down and get up so often, who wants to fiddle with laces?"

» **Small cooler with ice pack:** "You may not always have immediate access to a refrigerator for pumped breast milk, especially in the middle of the night!"

» **Small stuffed animals:** "The nurses will use them to prop up tubes, arms, legs—and even your baby."

» **Socks and hats:** "Calories are preserved by keeping the heat in."

» **Two-piece pajamas for your child:** "Pajamas with snaps and no feet. NO ZIPPERS! The lines and tubes will make zippers and footed jammies impossible."

» **Wet wipes**

TIPS TO PROMOTE INFANT DEVELOPMENT IN THE HOSPITAL

Samantha Butler, PhD, and Terra Lafranchi, MSN, RN, NP-C

The tips below were designed to promote your baby's development throughout their hospital stay. These tips may need to be changed based on your baby's medical status and their unique and changing individual needs. Your baby's bedside nurse and care team will help decide the best timing for you to try some of these ideas.

» **Try to create a quiet and calm environment for your baby to heal from surgery.** Lower voices, phone rings, music, TV and other noises next to your baby's bed. Also try to dim bright lights when possible.

» **Give your baby boundaries, like they had in the womb, so they feel support on all sides of their body.** Use rolled blankets as bumpers around your baby to support arms and legs. When possible, hold and place your baby on their side with their arms and legs tucked in. Bring soft blankets and soft stuffed animals to the bedside to support positioning and comfort.

» **Take your time when caring for your baby and take frequent breaks which will allow your baby to stay calm during care.** When your baby is over- stimulated, they may yawn, stick their tongue out, stretch out their arms and legs, and stretch out their fingers. These behaviors are good signals to pause and give your baby a break. Put your hands around your baby or hold your baby until they relax.

» **Hold your baby either in your arms or ideally on your chest and give skin-to-skin comforting when possible.** Your baby will feel more safe with your touch. There is nothing your baby would rather have than you supporting their care. Even when your baby needs to stay in their crib, gently touch or place your hands around them. Most babies are sensitive after surgery and like your hands placed on them or holding them with little movement. They often find petting or stroking over-stimulating. If your baby is stable, the time before surgery is a wonderful time to hold and cuddle your baby as much as possible because there may be several days after surgery when you may not be able to hold your baby.

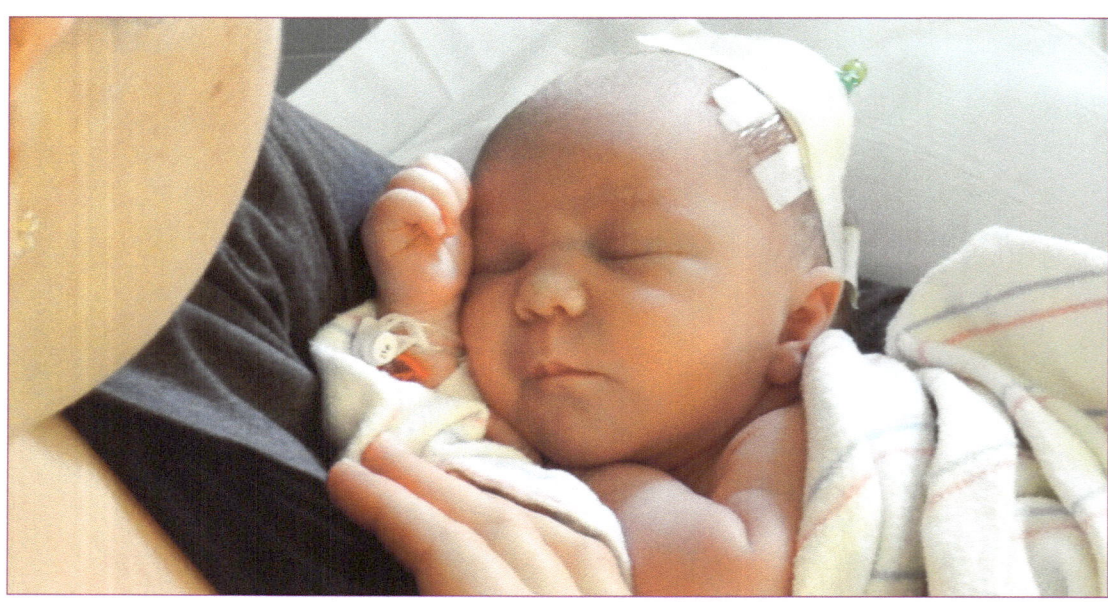

Kerri, holding and comforting baby Peter in the hospital

» **Offer your baby a pacifier during caregiving.** Most babies settle by sucking on a pacifier. They also enjoy sucking on their own fingers. You can help them bring their hands to their mouth.

» **Offer items to hold in their hands such as a soft blanket, stuffed animal, or your finger.**

» **Talk and sing to your baby in a soft voice.** Babies like to hear the voices of their parents. They are familiar with your voice from within the womb.

» **Leave a soft cloth that smells like you for your baby when you cannot be with them.** Babies know and enjoy the smell of their parents. You can tuck the cloth in your shirt for a few minutes before leaving it for your baby.

» **Read, sing, talk and make eye contact with your newborn baby to help with brain development.** The American Academy of Pediatrics and the Center for Media and Child Health strongly discourage television viewing for children younger than 2 years of age. Our hospital has books that you can borrow to read to your baby. Bring photographs of your family and drawings for soft decoration of your baby's crib.

» **As soon as medically possible, hold your baby during all feedings.** Feeding is a social activity, and babies enjoy being held during eating, even when taking in their food by a feeding tube.

» **Offer a pacifier during tube feedings so that your baby can start to learn that sucking leads to a full belly.** Sucking will also provide saliva which aides in digestion.

» **If possible, give breast milk for your baby.** Pumping is often needed to give breast milk to the baby after surgery. Most babies benefit from breast milk during their hospital stay.

» **Practice breastfeeding as soon as possible.** Allow your baby to "practice" breast-feeding even if they are not fully feeding by mouth. Practice breastfeeding by putting your baby in position to breastfeed, and allow your baby to nuzzle at the breast during skin-to-skin holding with mother.

» **Ask for a lactation consult as soon as possible, even before your baby is ready to feed by mouth.** Lactation is helpful in supporting the mother who is pumping.

Recommendations adapted from the developmental care guidelines. Als H., McAnulty G. Developmental care guidelines for use in the Newborn Intensive Care Unit. Boston: Boston Children's Hospital;1998.

YOUR FETAL CARDIOLOGY CARE CHECKLIST

☐ **Follow-up fetal echocardiogram** with Dr._____
in _____ weeks OR at_____ weeks pregnant.

☐ **Additional imaging or consults:**_____

☐ **Consider amniocentesis or other genetic testing.** If amniocentesis performed, we recommend FISH for 22q11.2 deletion (also referred to as DiGeorge Syndrome).

☐ **Please talk to your obstetrician about delivering closer to Boston Children's.** You may now be cared for by a high-risk obstetrician (also called a maternal-fetal medicine, or MFM, doctor) at the hospital where you will deliver. You should be cared for by your local OB until you have your first clinic visit with your Boston high-risk OB and you have made a plan for care. Your local OB and your Boston high-risk OB may decide to share your care so that you do not have to travel to Boston for all of your OB appointments. You will discuss delivery planning and when to relocate to Boston with your high-risk OB.

☐ **Please meet with the Neonatal ICU team at your delivery hospital.** The Neonatal ICU team will be present in the delivery room to help keep your baby stable and to help transfer your baby to the Cardiac ICU. The length of time that your baby stays in the Neonatal ICU before coming to Boston Children's ICU will depend on many factors that we will discuss with you.

☐ **Please tour the Cardiac ICU.** We have found that most families benefit from touring the Cardiac ICU before delivery. A tour of the CICU can be arranged to coincide with other appointments at Boston Children's Hospital or your Boston delivery hospital and will help to prepare you for your baby's care.

☐ **Please meet with the AFCC social worker.** Our social worker, Laurie Taylor, LICSW, is available to support families adjusting to the impact of the diagnosis, planning for the road ahead and struggling with making difficult decisions. She is also available to answer questions about travel, accommodations and resources. In addition, she also schedules tours of the Cardiac ICU and lactation consultations. You can reach Laurie at 617-355-3896 or laurie.olivertaylor@childrens.harvard.edu.

☐ **Learn about resources provided to you by hospital.** The Boston Children's Hospital Center for Families is available to help you and your family with any questions or concerns about care, the logistics of your hospital stay and anything else you may need. The Center for Families can be contacted at 617-355-6279. The center is located in the hospital lobby and you are encouraged to stop in at any time.

☐ **Call Patient Financial Services.** If you have questions about billing or insurance coverage please call: 617-355-3397.

☐ **Learn about family housing.** For Information about patient family housing, please call 617-919-3450. *Family housing rooms book up quickly-please make a reservation as soon as possible! You may make a reservation up to three months prior to your requested arrival date, so you can submit your application now.* Families often make a reservation from the time that they will arrive in Boston (before delivery) until about one month after their due date. This reservation may need to be longer or shorter based on your specific situation. You may also want to contact your insurance company to see if they might help with lodging and travel expenses.

☐ **Meet with a lactation specialist.** For many reasons, breast milk is valuable and important in the care of babies with congenital heart defects. If you are interested in breastfeeding and pumping breast milk for your baby, you will be able to meet with a lactation specialist before giving birth. Our lactation specialists are available to support you during pregnancy, after delivery and throughout your baby's hospitalization and care. Our lactation specialists can be reached at 617-355-2086.

☐ **Meet your fetal and pediatric cardiologist.** The cardiologist who performed your echocardiogram may not be your baby's cardiologist after birth. Ask who your pediatric cardiologist will be and if you can meet them prenatally and how to contact them with any questions or concerns. The name of your pediatric cardiologist is:_____.

☐ **Meet our cardiac geneticist.** If your baby has any other birth defects, or if you have a family history of pediatric heart problems, we suggest that you meet with a genetic counselor and our cardiac geneticist before or after your baby's birth.

☐	**It takes a village.** You are embarking on a complicated journey. Families do best when they accept available supports. As you prepare for your baby's arrival make a list of the things you may need help with (ie: feeding/walking the dog, childcare during delivery, rides for other children to school/activities, meals, errands, transportation, laundry, fundraising, emotional support, etc.). You will need help. Please ask for help and please accept help when it is offered to you. When people offer to help, give them a specific task.
☐	**Support is available.** There are a variety of emotions you may face during your pregnancy, the first hospitalization and as your child grows. As you build your support structure for this journey, consider whether it would be helpful to have a therapist accompany you on this difficult road. Our social worker can provide you with a local referral, if that would be helpful. If you need more support, please tell your cardiology team, social worker, obstetrician, or primary care physician. You are not alone.
☐	**Know your reliable sources of information.** Please visit the Boston Children's Hospital website for further information about your baby's diagnosis. Be careful about visiting other websites and parent blogs as this information is not always accurate or may not apply to your baby's diagnosis. Please call or email your cardiologist and our team with any questions or concerns. We would prefer that you reach out to us, rather than worry at home alone until your next appointment.
☐	**Choose a primary care pediatrician.** You will need to choose a pediatrician to care for your baby's routine health needs. The pediatrician should be close to your home. Before making your decision, ask about their comfort level and experience in caring for children with congenital heart defects. If you are having trouble locating the right doctor, ask us early so we can help.

NOTES:

NOTES:

www.ingramcontent.com/pod-product-compliance
Lightning Source LLC
Chambersburg PA
CBHW060833290526
45792CB00006BB/1914